this kind of child

K. Srilata is a poet, fiction writer, translator and academic. She was a writer in residence at Sangam House, India, Yeonhui Art Space, Seoul, and the University of Stirling, Scotland.

Srilata's novel *Table for Four* (Penguin) was longlisted in 2009 for the Man Asian Literary Prize. Her books include five collections of poetry, the latest of which, *The Unmistakable Presence of Absent Humans*, was published by Poetrywala, Mumbai. Srilata has also edited the anthologies *The Rapids of a Great River: The Penguin Book of Tamil Poetry* (Penguin), *Short Fiction from South India* (OUP), *All the Worlds Between: A Collaborative Poetry Project Between India and Ireland* (Yoda) and *Lifescapes: Interviews with Contemporary Women Writers from Tamilnadu* (Women Unlimited).

Formerly a professor of literature at IIT Madras, Srilata is now director of the Centre for Creative Writing and Translation at Sai University, Chennai. Srilata was recently awarded an IFA Arts Practice grant to work on a manuscript of poems based on the Mahabharata canon.

this kind of child

the 'disability' story

K. SRILATA

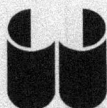

WESTLAND
NON·FICTION

First published by Westland Non-Fiction, an imprint of Westland Books, a division of Nasadiya Technologies Private Limited, in 2022

No. 269/2B, First Floor, 'Irai Arul', Vimalraj Street, Nethaji Nagar, Allappakkam Main Road, Maduravoyal, Chennai 600095

Westland, the Westland logo, Westland Non-Fiction and the Westland Non-Fiction logo are the trademarks of Nasadiya Technologies Private Limited, or its affiliates.

ISBN: 9789395767521

Typeset by SÜRYA, New Delhi

Printed at Nutech Print Services-India

CONTENTS

BOOK THREE: THE WHISPER OF
YOUR HEAD TILTING

BOOK FOUR: LOVE'S LABOUR

BOOK FIVE: SIBLINGS AND CHILDREN

BOOK SIX: CREATING ROADMAPS AND SPACES

BOOK SEVEN: YOU EXPERT WOMAN, YOU
Interleaved Stories | *K. Srilata*

Note on Terms Used

Throughout this book, I have used people-first language, preferring the terms 'persons with disabilities' or 'people with disabilities' to 'disabled' or 'disabled person'. This is in keeping with the belief that a person isn't a disability, a condition or a diagnosis. Rather, a person *has* a disability, a condition or a diagnosis. I have also avoided the use of the phrase 'special needs' because of the condescension that goes with its usage. Exceptions have been made, however, in the case of interviews and first-person accounts where people have sometimes chosen to use the word 'disabled', 'deaf', 'blind' or 'special needs' while referring to themselves or those they work with and care for.

Preface

When I started working on this manuscript, it was my daughter who was, in some senses, its protagonist. What eventually turned into this book was, at first, a series of interleaved short stories centred on the life of a child who doesn't fit the school system. These stories have remained part of the fabric of the text but I have placed them at the very end, their fictionality gesturing to the fact that the field I wandered into serendipitously and which now has me in its thrall is wide open, that to conclude a book like this is an impossibility. There is no way I could have stopped with those stories, for they were the stories of an entire universe of humans hidden in plain sight.

I am not the first to tell the disability story. Nor will I be the last. I have never identified as a person with a disability even though there are so many things my ageing body can no longer do. But equally, the thread that connects me to the community of persons with disabilities is less slender than it might appear. For I am the mother of a child who did not fit the school system, a child who was disabled by it. She was a child who made 'errors', 'mistakes' that the school system was unforgiving of. We were told by the principal of an alternative school that they could not possibly admit 'this kind of child'. My daughter went from being a child to 'this kind of child' in that one moment. This is the place from which I started to listen in on the larger story of the things we frame as 'disability', the systemic violence of institutions which fail human beings and punish them for inhabiting certain bodies, certain minds.

I also began to recognise in the 'disability' story, parts of myself and all the ways in which I am not completely 'able' or even 'independent'. This listening has brought me many gifts. I have learnt that disability is profoundly political, that it is heartbreakingly social. I have learnt about the hard, invisible and utterly fulfilling labour that is love and care. I have learnt what it means to report from the margins. I have learnt that stories are always bigger than they seem at first—bigger, wider and deeper. I have learnt that all stories have meeting points and that these meeting points have to do with inter-being.

This book has grown in an organic way to make space for the voices of persons with minds and bodies that are not 'neurotypical', the voices of those who care for them and teach them. Its scope has expanded to let in first-person accounts, interviews and short fiction. I have let in rather than kept out voices and people—there was no way not to, for they walked right in. These lines from Ruth Vanita's story 'Vision' featured in this book capture perfectly what I feel: 'Today, I saw a whole other world just a few steps away from where I live. How much I saw in a few minutes! There are more worlds to be seen—the worlds in me, worlds beyond me, new worlds being made, worlds that could be made. I have to make up for the years, the centuries, I have lived with limited vision.'

Between the time of this book's conception and now, my daughter has grown up. She is now an adult. She has survived the brutalities that underlie a school system built around the idea of competition and a very narrow definition of academic success, brutalities she describes in her essay 'Words Like Swords'. Dyslexia no longer defines who she is. She has a fledgling sense of herself. But she is no longer the book's sole protagonist.

Introduction

Towards an Understanding of the 'Disability' Story

There is an old Buddhist story with resonances for the disability story we are about to embark on. When Kisa Gautami, the wife of a wealthy man of Shravasti, the capital of Kosala, loses her only son, she is overcome by a great sorrow and nearly loses her mind. Following the advice of an old man, she meets the Buddha, who tells her: 'I can revive your child on one condition. Bring me four or five mustard seeds from any family in which there has never been a death.' Gautami sets out to do his bidding, wandering desperately from house to house—only to find that there isn't a single one which has not experienced death. This, to her, is a profound lesson on mortality, the fact that death is *everywhere*.

To look for a body that has never experienced disability, or for people who have never been touched by the disability experience, is akin to Kisa Gautami's search for a family that had never suffered death. Chances are that we all know someone who has a disability. This person may have a disability from birth, may have acquired a disability later due to an illness or accident, or thanks to the ubiquitous process of ageing. This disability may be visible and obvious, or not. Our own bodies may have become, at various points, the sites of a disability—due either to the natural process of ageing or an accident. There is another issue we might want to keep in mind when it comes to thinking about people with disabilities. Sometimes, we hear that someone has 'outgrown', 'overcome' or 'compensated for' a disability. But for every such 'positive' account, there are also people who can't or don't 'outgrow' or 'overcome' their disabilities. Given our culture's preference for 'success' stories, the only people with disabilities we want to hear about or hear from are the ones who have 'made it' in some way. The narrative of overcoming is, of course, a powerful one, and not to be discounted. However, this should not be the *only* narrative we pay heed to. What we should be asking ourselves is: What of the 'non-successes'? What of their lives? What are the cracks through which they have fallen? How have they been failed? What value do their lives hold inherently? What of the lives of those who live with disabling pain that prevents them from leading a full life?

The thing about disability is that it could happen to anyone. Age or accidents could disable us in some way. We are unlikely to inhabit able bodies throughout life. Our bodies and our minds are in a constant state of flux. We just don't see it. And so, we tend to think of disability as another planet of experience altogether, something that *has not, will not* and *should not* happen to us.

Disability is a no-man's land. Mainstream medicine, by its very nature, is focused on the 'treatable' and the 'curable'. Chronic illnesses, pain and disabilities are often impossible to 'treat' or 'fix'. Poorly understood and poorly researched, these bodily experiences become nobody's babies and tend to be locked away in tiny silos such as 'special schools' and the private space of the home. They are experiences no one wants to talk about. The body with a disability is a suffering body, a body we would do anything to avoid. And when I use the word body, I am also, of course, referring to the mind, which is inseparable from the body. But the good news is that the work of creating the vocabulary to describe and enhance the understanding of this experience is happening. Much of this vocabulary is being developed by people with disabilities or by people closely associated with them. Spoon theory* is one example, as is the term 'specific learning disability'.

Self-representation is critical to the disability narrative. Especially given the extent to which disability is mis-represented—even ridiculed—in mainstream culture.

As Susan Wendell points out in her essay 'Towards a Feminist Theory of Disability', people with disabilities learn what many, perhaps most, 'able-bodied people' do not want to know about the suffering caused by the body. Bodily suffering and the inability to control the body are feared, pitied and despised. But what is the nature of the learning that accrues from this apparently negative experience of the body? What are the understandings, the language that comes from that space? What does it mean to live as a person with disabilities in a world that is overwhelmingly ableist? How does one navigate everyday and not-so-everyday moments in a world that is not set up for one? What do people with disabilities want for themselves? This book asks and attempts to respond to some of these questions.

The larger universe of persons with disabilities includes

---

* In a blog titled 'The Spoon Theory', Christine Miserandino describes how she showed her friend what it's like to have lupus, an autoimmune disease characterised by fatigue, fever and joint pain. While sitting at a diner, Miserandino handed her friend twelve spoons, each representing a unit of energy. She then asked her friend to describe the typical activities of a day. Miserandino took away a spoon for every single task: showering, getting dressed with painful joints, standing on a train. Skipping lunch would cost a spoon, too. When the spoons were gone, it meant there was barely energy to do anything else. This idea of quantifying energy as spoons, and the idea that people with chronic disease only get a handful of spoons each day, is what is known as 'spoon theory'. It is now part of the lingo of autoimmune disease.

persons who love and care for them. The lives of the latter are just as easily overlooked. The labour of care and love are not easily monetised. This work, then, is usually unaccounted for and this ties in with the fact that, most often, it is women who take on caregiving. For instance, in most cases involving children with disabilities, it is the mothers who assume the role of caregivers, often at great personal and professional costs, which they may not recognise as costs for it is love that drives their work. By a peculiar sleight of hand, then, caregiving itself becomes feminised (even when it is a man who is doing it). This further feeds the perception that it is not 'real' work. But this labour must be seen, acknowledged and valued. And we need a language in which to do that. My interviews with Waheeda, Nimi, Swati and Mamtha bear this out.

Caregiving hours are not billable. They cannot be easily explained or described. They cannot easily be accounted for. One of the tasks I set myself was to inch closer to that accounting. Consequently, this book has also become a book about the labour of care, which is really expertise of a crucial kind, a symbiotic knowledge economy that works in fascinating ways. For the work of caring or caregiving is mainly about figuring out what works and setting up an informal community of expertise. This is perhaps most obvious from my conversation with Mamtha, the mother of a young man with DAMP syndrome.

The more people I met, the more stories I heard, my field of enquiry grew, became an ever-widening circle. There was no way not to include the stories of the children and siblings of persons with disabilities. And so, an interview with Chetna and first-person accounts by V.R. Krishnan, Aniruddha and Karthika, too, find a place in this book

This book is an attempt to place centre-stage a diverse range of disability narratives—narratives of recovery alongside narratives of chronic suffering, narratives of persons with disability alongside narratives of their caregivers, parents and educators, of hidden disabilities and of visible ones, of disabilities at birth versus acquired disabilities. It intersperses fiction with autobiographical accounts and interviews/ conversations, as a way of offering multiple entry points and perspectives on disability.

It is my hope that this book will help us see that while we may not identify as persons with disabilities, while we may believe that we not have experienced disability first-hand, we are far more connected to those with officially diagnosed disabilities than we may suspect. The disability narrative is not some alien narrative that is out there. Disability is not, contrary to what we believe, another planet. It is part of the human experience and we have no choice but to engage with it, to articulate a fuller theory.

As I have already indicated, disability is used here as an umbrella term that is designed to include rather than exclude: people who self-identify as people with disabilities and/or have been diagnosed or certified as 'disabled', people with 'milder' or less obvious disabilities that do not 'count' as disabilities, people who may appear 'disabled' to others but who do not experience themselves as such (certain deaf communities in the USA are a case in point), people with hidden disabilities, such as learning disabilities or certain forms of mental illnesses, people who are born with a disability and therefore may be considered to have a 'stable' disability, people who acquire disabilities later in life due to an illness, accident or ageing, people whose disabilities may have been triggered or caused by their social environments or by adverse experiences such as abandonment in infancy, people with multiple disabilities and people whose disabilities intersect with other factors such as gender, class, caste, race, nationality and cultural background.[*]

Increasingly, there has been a move away from the medical model of disability, which tends to understand disability in the very narrow sense of 'impairment', and the body itself as something to be controlled by medical experts, to the social model of disability, developed in Britain in the 1970s. In 1976, the Union of the Physically Impaired Against Segregation published its *Fundamental Principles of Disability*, which distinguished impairment from disability:

In our view it is society which disables physically impaired people. Disability is something which is imposed on top of our impairments, by the way we are unnecessarily isolated and excluded from full participation in society.[†]

The medical model of disability when applied to psychiatric illness, for instance, is especially problematic, given the powerful hold that the psychiatrist has over patients and the often coercive practices of confinement in mental hospitals and psychiatric wards.

The social model refutes the traditional model of disability as personal misfortune or as something to be 'fixed' and 'treated', recasting it instead in terms of social oppression. This model has birthed a rights-based advocacy approach to disability. Activists and intellectuals interested in the disability question have pointed out, however, that quite often pain and real physical or mental agony needs medical intervention

---

[*] Meri Danquah's memoir *Willow Weep for Me*, for instance, is a powerful exploration of what it means to be a Black woman with depression.

[†] Lennard Davis (ed.), *The Disability Studies Reader* (2nd Edition), New York: Routledge, 2006, p. 287.

and that there has to be equal access to medical help for all people with disabilities.

Where all these debates lead to most urgently is perhaps the need to understand things from the ground up, to see that people with disabilities have their own ways of knowing and that their caregivers and educators learn on the job, figuring out innovative, experience-based caregiving or pedagogical 'solutions' that are not to be found in the pages of any textbook or manual. Especially significant is the idea of interdependence (rather than a narrowly defined 'independence') as value and virtue when it comes to understanding the disability experience. People do not and must not lead totally separate and thereby 'independent' lives. That's not the point of human experience. Nothing drives this point home more than the stories in this book, in which lives are richly intertwined with each other, long past the onset of official 'adulthood'.

I hope to offer a multi-perspectival understanding of what the disability experience really means, its emotional as well as imagined truth, both to people with disabilities as well as to those closely associated with them. The disability experience is not so much about a non-normative body or a mind that needs fixing. It is a complex world of human experience driven by its own logic, imagination and intelligence, a world that suffers from being neatly boxed. It deserves to be arrived at via multiple routes—the imaginative as well as the 'real'. This explains the somewhat unusual structure of the book—its attempt to combine the fictional with the non-fictional.

This Kind of Child is as much about ability, love, care and responsibility as it is about disability. It asks the questions: What does it mean to love and accept yourself or someone else fully? What abilities does it call forth? What new ways of being human?

A Note on the Structure of the Book

Certain themes and narratives came up repeatedly across the three broad genres represented here—personal essays, interviews or conversations, and short fiction. These were clearly part of a larger conversation surrounding 'disability', pieces of a puzzle that fit together. Therefore, an entirely genre-wise classification of the material in this book made little sense. With the exception of the inter-leaved stories at the very end, I have organised the material thematically and not genre-wise. The book comprises the following seven mini 'books', each designed to offer a particular perspective or dwell on a certain idea:

- Book One—School: The perspective of young people whose learning styles don't fit the school system.
- Book Two—On Our Terms: The perspective of persons who identify as 'disabled'.
- Book Three—The Whisper of Your Head Tilting: The idea of seeing and sight.
- Book Four—Love's Labour: The perspective of parents of children with disabilities.
- Book Five—Siblings and Children: The perspective of siblings and children of persons with disabilities.
- Book Six—Creating Roadmaps and Spaces: The perspective of those who teach or offer support services for persons with disabilities.
- Book Seven—You Expert Woman, You: Inter-leaved short stories written by me about a child with dyslexia and her mother.

Books one through six are set off by a note or commentary. Readers will find plenty of echoes, cross-references and connections between these books and that, of course, is the idea. The books are, after all, meant to be read together, even though they work in standalone fashion.

In some cases, an essay or a conversation could just as easily have been placed in another book. For instance, I decided to place the interview with Amaresh Gopalakrishnan in Book Six—Creating Roadmaps and Spaces. Amaresh is involved in sign language research and training. He also happens to be a CODA, a child of deaf adults. So, the interview belongs equally in Book Five—Siblings and Children.

BOOK ONE

School

Note

The preamble to the United Nations Convention on the Rights of Persons with Disabilities recognises that disability results from the *'interaction* [emphasis mine] between persons with impairments and attitudinal and environmental barriers that hinders their full and effective participation in society on an equal basis with others'. These barriers come in many guises. Some of them we have now learnt to see as barriers for persons with physical impairments— buildings without ramps or lifts that people with mobility challenges will find difficult or impossible to access, or traffic lights that a person with visual impairment would find impossible to navigate. But educational institutions, which we have been taught to see as enabling, can be profoundly disabling too. Schools, colleges, other educational institutions, pedagogical practices and mechanisms for evaluation, all of these can potentially become insurmountable barriers for some kinds of learners—as insurmountable as stairs for someone who is mobility challenged. This leads to the shunting of a young person from one institution to another, in a desperate search for a solution. Even those educational institutions that claim to be inclusive can prove to be difficult places for anyone who is differently wired. More young people fall through the cracks of these institutions than one realises and for the ones who survive them, the survival is often a result of superhuman effort and family support. It also typically comes at a huge psychological cost. There is a price to pay, for these systems can break and scar you in insidious ways.

The pieces that follow are, in part, reflections on how school can turn certain impairments (and even just certain ways in which a person's mind is wired) into disabilities. In what ways do schools and colleges disable our young?

Words Like Swords

Ananya Kambhampati

Ananya Kambhampati is a third-year undergraduate student at Christ University, Bengaluru, where she is pursuing a triple major in Western music, psychology and literature.

From kindergarten till about the middle of grade six, I went to a small Montessori school in Chennai. Some of my best memories were forged there. I made some amazing friends in this school, friends with whom I am still in touch—like my best friend Kalyani. I vividly remember not particularly liking her in the beginning but now she happens to be one of my closest friends! My teachers there were extremely kind and they cared about me. All except for one who, as it happened, also taught my brother. I am different from my brother in many ways and I also learn differently from him. This particular teacher would insist that I should emulate my brother and be the same sort of student that he was. This was also the time I realised I actually found reading and writing somewhat more difficult than other children. I needed help and time to catch up with my peers. But it was difficult to find the time and to access the help I required, given my school schedule.

When I was in the sixth grade, my parents and I agreed that I would be homeschooled for a year. I left school half way through the academic year. I was to miss that Montessori school for years afterwards, though especially the amazing friends I acquired during my years there.

Homeschooling proved to be a good break for me. That

year gave me the time not just to get comfortable with reading and writing, but also to explore other interests and hobbies. During this time, I went to a resource centre for homeschooled children. This was a wonderful experience. I managed to make some friends in this centre as well. But after that one year, I was ready to return to school.

I was then admitted to a small, fairly new school. Not to brag, but I quickly became Miss Popular and got a huge circle of friends. I also had the best class teacher ever, right through the three years that I was there. She taught me to always be myself and love who I was and not care about how others perceive me. I was even elected sports captain and subsequently, head girl of the school.

I hit a rough patch in grade ten, when I had a falling out with a classmate who had also been a close friend of mine. This got me very upset and part of me shut down and stopped trusting people. That year felt like a living hell, but I got myself out of it because of my brother. He didn't have to sit with me and talk to me for hours on end, but he always let me know that no matter what happened, he would be there for me. This gave me the strength to get through the year. Trusting people is still a problem for me but I am working on it.

At the end of grade ten, I switched to another school that offered psychology, a subject I was keen on. I didn't make many friends during the first eight months of my time in this new school. I spent much of grade eleven alone and unhappy.

I have never fared well academically, never been a topper. But this has not affected me any more than the insults I have received for scoring poorly. Sometimes, teachers labelled me an idiot, declaring that I must have a low IQ. What people do not realise about dyslexia or other learning difficulties is that they affect a person as much or even more than physical disabilities. The insults that were hurled at me for being 'bad' at things that others my age had mastered easily were like swords through my heart. I am now in grade twelve and though this still happens, I am working on ignoring these insults and focusing instead on my goal to become a psychologist.

A few things have gotten me through these tough times: my family, my two best friends—Akriti and Kalyani—and my music. Akriti has been in my life since I was a year old, and Kalyani since the age of five. They have supported me through some of the toughest times and have celebrated my happiest moments. My family has always allowed me to explore the world. They have caught me when I have fallen and taught me how to get back on my feet. Music has also been a huge part of my life. I started singing at the age of four and found that it helped me a lot during my difficult tenth grade year, as much as it has during other trying times. I am happiest when I am with my family, my best friends or my music, because they bring out the best in me.

In the future, I see myself as a music therapist. I am aware of just how much music has helped me and I would like to use music to help others, to make them feel better about life. My dream is to be a successful music therapist and have three big dogs.

What the Children of Sankalp Say

Snippets from a Conversation

What follows are snippets from an informal chat I had with a group of four sixteen-year-old students of Sankalp, an open school based in Chennai, for children with Specific Learning Disabilities (SLD). All four children are 'refugees', in a sense, from the harsh environment of mainstream schools, schools that they left in order to join Sankalp.

In my old school, they used to ignore me.

In the school I went to before I came to Sankalp, they didn't treat me well. I had no problem with friends though. Once, there was some kind of competition—some activity. My teacher told me not to participate even though I was all set for it. She said I could participate later but didn't call on me at all. When I asked her why, she said it was 'just like that'. I went home crying. When my mother saw me crying, she said, 'Enough is enough. You don't go to that school.' It was the middle of the term. I was in class four at the time.

In my old school, my teachers always said I was not good at academics. They told my mother that I should not participate in sports, even though I was good at sports. They said, 'Let him study. He is not capable.' My parents didn't know I had dyslexia then.

In the old school, my teacher would read my answers out in front of the entire class. If my spellings or my answers were wrong, she would make doubly sure to read the whole thing out. After that, my classmates would look at me as though I was weird. I remember I was hanging around once. I wasn't playing or anything but I happened to be really sweaty. My teacher assumed that I had been playing when I was supposed to be studying and marched me off to the principal's office. They gave me a 'remark' for that. After that, the others started looking at me differently. There was this boy who was an artist. He used to teach me drawing. The others would ask him why he was being my friend. They never played with me. Both the teachers and students at my old school used to judge me.

I left my old school because my teachers were extremely strict. I was a very slow learner. I took time to understand things. They used to hit me, make me stand outside the class.

In my old school, they would stop me from participating in extracurricular activities because I wasn't a good student. At Sankalp, I get many opportunities to participate in these activities. I am good at giving speeches in English. I play the keyboard.

At Sankalp, they forgive me many things! I am good at making music. I love music, EDM especially. I am good at squash and cycling.

In my old school, my physical education teacher liked me because I was good at swimming. I had even got some medals. But my teachers always said, 'He is not good at academics. Let him focus on his lessons.' So, I quit swimming. In that school, none of the teachers knew I was good at drawing. It was only after coming to this school that I started going for drawing competitions.

I am really scared of math. But at Sankalp, I am learning practical math.

I have challenges in writing. I have started writing a little now—at Sankalp. I will get a scribe.

In this school, I write when I am in the mood, when I am happy.

I just get bored with writing sometimes.

I have trouble remembering big words. I make spelling mistakes. I remember the whole story but forget the names of places, people, etc.

I am preparing for the SAT exam. I want to become an English professor. I am aiming to join Cambridge.

I am looking at a career as a DJ.

I am thinking of doing visual communication.

I am going to be a music producer.

When I tell people I am dyslexic, they don't understand. They think we are special children; they think this is some big disability or a big problem.

Many people don't know what Sankalp is, what NIOS* is.

I just tell them Sankalp is a special school where they help children who have difficulty learning. Some people think it is a school for children who can't see or hear. I tell them it is a just a regular, normal school where they teach slowly and take care of us.

When I was in the old school, my parents thought that I was not willing to study. I didn't know what to do. My father used to say that everyone can study and do well academically. He changed his view only after we met a doctor. That is when he understood dyslexia.

Schools shouldn't be rude to children like us. They shouldn't tell other children not to socialise or play with us. Sometimes, in front of other parents, they treat our parents badly. That's why my father used to get angry with me when I was in the other school.

---

* The National Institute of Open Schooling which allows homeschooled children, adult learners and those who want to learn at their own pace to study and take a recognised school leaving exam when they are ready.

At my old school, they used to punish us, threaten the other children that they too would become like us if they didn't study.

The teachers in my old school would tell us we had no future, that we would amount to nothing; we would never become lawyers or policemen.

When people tell me dyslexic people can't do anything, I tell them about Albert Einstein!

There's also a well-known YouTuber, gamer and animator who is dyslexic. Those who didn't want to know him before now want his autograph!

We should always say positive things to children. That energy flow works!

Air Hostess Dreams

An Interview with Diya Sankar

Diya Sankar is a twenty-four-year-old with a hearing impairment. Currently a trainee at a star hotel in Hyderabad, she graduated from college with a degree in tourism and travel. Her parents, Shoba and Sankaravadivelu (conversations with whom feature elsewhere in this book), learnt that she was hearing-impaired when she was two years of age. Subsequently, she received intensive speech therapy in Chennai. Her mother, Shoba, was present right through our conversation and occasionally participated in it.

Srilata: Tell me about yourself, your life in school before you joined college.

Diya: I don't remember much about Bala Vidyalaya.

Srilata: How about your friends? Do you remember them?

Diya: Sanjana, Karen, Roshan, Megha, Sangeeth—these were my batchmates. We were in the same class. We all moved to different schools. I moved to Vidya Mandir, Mylapore. I was there till sixth standard. I didn't like maths. So, I left that school. My mom put me in another school, an international school. Then, from there, I moved to Ananya Learning Centre. You could learn at your pace there. They didn't force you. I liked computers, social science ... Public exams were held in tenth standard. They used to test us on a few chapters. They would let us repeat these tests. So, I was doing well. For my tests, I learnt things by rote. I had a good memory. I passed the public exam.

Srilata: You did well too ...

Diya: Yes, my teachers used to like me a lot. After that, I joined Ethiraj College. Actually, I wanted to join a co-ed college, like the Madras Christian College, but my mom wanted me to join a girls' college.

Shoba: But the Madras Christian College didn't offer travel and tourism, which was the course you wanted.

Diya: I had some problems with my friends in Ethiraj. They tended to blame me for everything. That was not fair.

Shoba: She didn't enjoy Ethiraj.

Srilata: Were the class sizes big?

Diya: But the teachers were good. Now I have to find a job, my mom said I should look for a job. We have to attend a wedding in a few days but after that I have to start looking for work.

Srilata: What would have made you happier at school and at college?

Diya: In college, there were just too many students. The classrooms were packed.

Shoba: Were your classmates friendly?

Diya: They were.

Shoba: Is it that there were no other children like you?

Diya: There were other children like me in the evening college. I always used to sit in the front row. But sometimes the teachers would say something and I would find it difficult to follow. Some children had scribes.

Shoba: The college had many visually impaired children.

Srilata: What would you like to do more than anything else? You are interested in fashion, aren't you?

Diya: My interest in dressing up is thanks to my mom. I like to go out. I want to go to America. My favourite cities are New York, London and Singapore.

Srilata: What kind of work are you looking for?

Diya: I would like to work as an air hostess. But you have to be able to hear well and understand in order to be employed as one. When [passengers] speak, you may not be able to understand. Maybe I will do something else involving computers—learn something new and then maybe I will go forward. If they give me an opportunity, I will work at the airport.

Srilata: Is there anything else you would like to say?

Diya: I love my parents. I will always be thankful to them!

Beyond Sameness

Dhaatri Vengunad Menon

Dhaatri Vengunad Menon is a visual storyteller who enjoys painting and cartooning. She is currently pursuing a course in children's book illustration and hopes to work towards a world that is more accepting of differences.

Dyslexia isn't just about not being able to write fast enough or neatly enough. It is also about being different, perceiving things differently and sometimes reacting differently to situations as compared to others. It means that the ideologies we believe in may be different. For instance, many of my friends with dyslexia do not believe in competing with others. They are kinder and believe that the world should have space for lots of different kinds of talents. This is generally different from the mainstream ideology that I have seen in most schools. This may be because people with dyslexia are labelled as 'being different', or even 'being disabled'. That experience of being bullied openly, and many times covertly, may be the reason we don't believe in win–lose situations, where one person wins and the others lose.

Today, everyone wants to be the same, to look the same and think the same. However, when you go to an event, everyone wants to be the star of the event and the centre of attraction by being different. This is logic that I have never understood. Why expect sameness and homogeneity when there can be heterogeneity? Why can't there be space for people who are different, for people who do things differently? When will we stop looking down on people who are different from us—be it based on thought, dress, religion, caste or academic abilities?

Socially, I have had many difficult and troubling experiences. I have even had parents of my friends advise me about how important it is to behave the same, dress the same and merge with my peers if I wish to be accepted at birthday parties and other social events. Maybe society feels threatened by people who think differently. My own family, however, has encouraged me to be myself and to think for myself. This has helped me and I have learnt to let go of hurtful memories and of the hurtful things people have said. Here, I must say that many of us who have been labelled as 'dyslexic' have the ability to think abstractly, are highly creative and imaginative, terribly funny and have strengths that may not be related to books and the written word.

People with dyslexia face an ongoing struggle to fit into the Indian education system. There is very little space for 'difference'. While the system definitely 'moulds' us, it does so in a way where every product has to be more or less the same. Then, the best of the same are rewarded. I have tried to chop off parts of me that are too different to merge in with the structure. But that, again, is too painful. So, it is a balance that I have had to strike to survive the system while remaining true to myself. What is lacking is a bridge in the system for these two extreme groups of sameness and differences. In the last couple of years, I have decided to be open about the fact that I have dyslexia and say it when I think the need arises. The reactions from the people around are many—some are unable to believe me and treat it like a lie. They feel that if someone speaks well, their writing and reading will also be perfect. Others treat me with sympathy—something I don't need, because it is *not* a misfortune to be dyslexic. Yet others (mainly teachers) think that I am hiding behind a condition and finding excuses for my laziness. I can assure you that people with dyslexia struggle with a lot of tasks and work a lot more than the average smarty.

If all schools and colleges allowed students to use laptops, speech-to-text devices, audio recordings or videos of lessons, many of us would not have to struggle so much. If all tests did not have to be written fast and in a given time, and some of them were drawings or oral tests, I would have found lots more time for the things that I am really interested in (like painting and poetry) and I would not have had to think of myself as 'inferior' to the student next to me just because I write slower. But then, the system is still a long way off from that model.

Sometimes, a stroke of sunlight in the darkness can mean everything to someone. I am thankful to the teachers who have encouraged me and held my hand through my school days. Most of them were from the Remedial Learning Centre. The master who included me in the band, the Learning Centre head who patiently and quietly insisted every day that it is great to be different and believed in me, the teachers who would put aside their red pens to mark my papers in blue— you are the sunshine. I used to think that my dyslexia would go away some time in the future, perhaps when I turned twenty. I used to think that life would, at some point, be a little less difficult. But the thing is, I am twenty now and the difficulties haven't really gone away.

But I am coming to see it all as a good thing, as a blessing—to be different.

BOOK TWO

On Our Terms

Note

The move away from the 'charity' model to the model of 'legitimate rights' has meant a seismic shift in thinking about disability. For persons with disabilities, the right to education, livelihood, independent living, self-determination, love or sexual expression are not automatically granted. They are hard-won and usually involve years of painful negotiations with mainstream structures and systems, both within the domestic, familial space and outside of it.

We slip easily into thinking of persons with disabilities as people in need of help. This default model of 'charity' is deeply flawed, for help and charity are necessitated mostly by an absence of institutional and systemic support for persons with disabilities. It is this absence that impoverishes the life of a person with disability, making self-determination an impossibility. In the charity model, it is the person with the disability who comes to be seen as the 'problem', as 'helpless', as needing care, sympathy and protection. In many ways, this model, relying as it does on charity and benevolence, can end up justifying the exclusion of persons with disabilities from the mainstream. On the other hand, the disability rights model perceives disability as an important dimension of human culture and is accepting of diversity and difference. It questions practices such as the segregation and institutionalisation of persons with disabilities.

Rights advocacy and activism that stem from within the community of persons with disabilities are extremely valuable and instructive in this respect. This said, as Rajiv Rajan, a disability rights activist points out in an interview featured in this book, not everyone from within the community of persons with disabilities is an activist. Nor should we require them to be. Like everyone else, persons with disabilities vary in their ability to articulate experience, to advocate for themselves and for others. And what of people like Gayathri, for whom speech and communication is a challenge? For theirs too are voices that we need to hear. As are the voices of people like Kim, who 'came out' as a person with a disability and for whom receiving care was something she had to learn to be less prickly about. For isn't this all equally about inter-being? The more I spoke to people with disabilities and those designated—officially or unofficially—as their 'caregivers', what emerged for me is the profound emotional connections between the two groups and the fact that their lives are mutually enriched by each other. And who is to say who 'depends' on whom and, indeed, isn't human interdependence of great value?

When I Became a Mother

Kristen Witucki

Kristen Witucki is a blind author, editor, teacher and mentor who lives in the north-eastern United States. She is the author of a fiction book for emerging adolescent readers, *The Transcriber*, a novel, *Outside Myself*, and several non-fiction articles. She lives with her husband, James Simmons, who is also blind, and her three sighted children: Langston (9), Noor (4) and Karuna (1).

'I didn't know she was coming,' the nurse told my sighted friend as she helped me into the soon-to-be-blood-soaked hospital gown. 'No one told me about this.' Was 'this' my blindness or the baby or both? She was right; the nurse hadn't been expecting me and I had not met her before. On my hospital tour, it was nurse Evelyn I had met. She had told me about a competent blind mother she knew and who, she assured me, would help me get a handle on mothering. Unfortunately for me, Langston had chosen to be born on Evelyn's day off.

'We took the tour and talked to several people here,' my friend, Suzanne, answered calmly.

'But I didn't know,' the nurse said, reminding us that we had not, in fact, talked to every single person in that massive hospital, emphasising the *I*, as if she alone had the power to usher or withhold my baby from the world.

Admissions couldn't find me in the computer, even though I had mailed in all of the paperwork early, and an administrative assistant asked me a few questions, basic pieces of information like my name and birth date, which I could ordinarily have answered with 100 per cent accuracy. But now, thanks to the waves of pain, which seemed to be crashing over each other with no beginning and no end, I found myself unable to utter a word.

The nurse checked me, and I thought, 'Please clear me for an epidural so I can talk.'

'She's nine and a half centimetres gone,' the nurse said, sounding impressed for the first time. 'She's ready to have the baby.'

Apparently, I was having the type of labour which only happens in made-for-TV movies. Except, in those movies, the blind person is never the woman having the baby.

So, as I struggled against the worry that the nurse wouldn't allow me to take my baby home, my son tried to exit, but he couldn't quite get it right. People connected several heart monitors to us and his heartbeat sounded slow and steady like mine. Although I couldn't spell my name out loud, I was suddenly telling the nurse, 'I think his heart rate is down.'

'It slows down during labour,' the nurse reassured me.

Then a male doctor entered and said, 'Kristen, are you listening? The heart rate is down.' (*Hadn't I just said that?*) 'If you can't get the baby out in the next fifteen minutes, we will need to do a C-section.'

I nodded.

The doctor explained that I would need to alert him when a contraction started and to push through it. I would feel one and manage to grind out an 'Okay' before pushing. My husband told me, 'You're doing great,' and I thought, 'How do you know? You can't see any of this!' I pushed and moaned and the doctor pulled with a vacuum and after a couple of tries, my son's head emerged. Then, with the next push, he slid out to someone ... not to me. Then he was gone ... but just to the other side of the room, my friend explained, as the doctor gave me some medication to survive being patched back together. Eventually, Suzanne said, reminding them, 'Will you give her the baby?'

They didn't hesitate, at least perceptibly. They handed me the baby, wrapped in a coarse hospital-issue blanket. I was holding my son. The blanket made him, for them, just like any other baby. Only later would I come to know him as the most beautiful creature, as *my* most beautiful creature: the protrusions of his shoulder blades beneath the slight ripple of his skin; the bones of his spine, each one as distinct as the beads on a necklace; the soft down of his hair; his piano hands opening and closing like mussel shells, moving foggily at times to block his path to my breast.

I was released from the hospital, but Langston had to return to the NICU due to jaundice. The NICU nurses asked me questions. How would I take the baby's temperature? Could I tell time? Did I have relatives living close by who would help? But these nurses seemed much nicer than that nurse I had met on the day of the delivery, the nurse who would rather I hold my baby inside myself. When I admitted to one NICU nurse that I hadn't totally figured out how to measure medicine, she suggested that the pharmacist could help by measuring it out ahead of time. I learnt later that I could buy droppers of different sizes, but I appreciated her willingness to help. For three days, as Langston's bilirubin returned to normal and they completed observations, I slept and healed, pumped milk and delivered it to the hospital. We worried. Would they let him go? My relatives and friends helpfully surrounded us, cocooned us, so that my advocacy efforts were minimal as I recovered. And eventually, they did release Langston, thinking, perhaps, that we were his parents only on paper, that we were not his actual caregivers. Caregivers, after all, were not supposed to be blind.

After a few days, my mom left us, with many cooked meals and everything organised, alone as a family to figure things out on our own. However, whenever we needed to bring the baby to the doctor, she always materialised. As long as she was there, I knew no one would question our legitimacy as parents. She wasn't able to go to our three-month appointment, but my good friend, Nancy, who was planning to visit anyway, assured me she could take us.

On the morning of the appointment, she called me, her voice a frog's croak. She had a cold, she said, and the roads around her were flooded. She probably shouldn't take us.

It was too late to reschedule the appointment. I called a cab, buckled Langston into his car seat, placed the backpack on my back, picked up the car seat, unfolded my cane, walked to the apartment door and opened it, walked outside, put the car seat down briefly so I could lock the apartment, picked up the seat, opened the main building door and guided the baby through it and down the steps so he wouldn't fall or be slammed by the door, and shuffled out to the cab. Then I opened the door, shoved the car seat over as far as I could and folded my cane and slid in beside it. When we reached the office, I climbed out of the cab with the seat, unfolded the cane, placed the seat on the ground next to me and called the office to ask if someone could help me get Langston and my stuff upstairs. The receptionist assured me effusively that this was not a problem and came to my aid. I worried that she was too effusive.

I prepared myself for an invisible wall in the cubicle sliding open to reveal an entourage of people with paper, informing me that I was officially not qualified to take care of my son.

A lone doctor walked through the door an eternity later, nonchalantly examined Langston, asked me about tummy time and my plans to start solids and pronounced him healthy. Then she left me alone with my baby. I was free to take him home.

As a new mother, I felt the same rocky emotions as other new mothers: deeply abiding joy and love, fear and worry that I wasn't doing enough or was doing it wrong, social isolation and, sometimes, even boredom with the never-ending cycle of feed, change, sleep, repeat. But the doctor's nonchalant acknowledgement of Langston and me as a viable dyad obliterated, for a moment, that complexity. I simply felt the relief of being considered 'normal', free to take Langston home.

A Question of Human Rights

A Conversation with Rajiv Rajan and Dheepakh P.S.

Rajiv Rajan is the executive director of Ektha, an organisation that advocates for the rights of persons with disabilities. He was formerly the coordinator of the Chennai-based NGO Vidya Sagar's Disability Law Unit, and continues to be associated with them. Rajiv has a PG diploma in human rights from the Indian Institute of Human Rights, New Delhi, with a specialisation in child rights and women's rights. He has been part of the disability rights movement for twenty-five years.

Dheepakh P.S. is currently serving as senior sub-editor of the Sports Desk at *The Hindu* and is a cricket buff and a sports enthusiast. He holds an honorary post in Ektha and is a founder-trustee and board member.

Srilata: Tell me about your early years before you came to Vidya Sagar.

Rajiv: My early years were spent sitting at home. I could read Malayalam, which is my mother tongue. I could do mathematics—multiplication, addition, division and subtraction. I was taught by my mother and my grandmother. My immediate family consists of my mother, my father (who passed away ten years ago), and me. My parents were very supportive.

Dheepakh: I joined Vidya Sagar in 1990, when I was four. My mother was a speech therapist here. Rajiv was my super-senior. He was the first to be integrated into a mainstream school.

Rajiv: Dheepakh's mother used to take classes for me.

Srilata: How did Vidya Sagar change things for you?

Rajiv: It was a totally different atmosphere. I took some time to adjust to it because, to be frank, I had until then never been exposed to a place where people around me drooled and so on. So, all those things had an impact. I couldn't eat for two or three days. It was that bad. But I recovered after a while. However, I did find it difficult to face the outside world.

Srilata: In what way?

Rajiv: People on the streets would stare at me. They would look at me as though I were an animal or a strange person from a different planet.

Dheepakh: They consider us aliens!

Srilata: Tell me about your experiences in mainstream school.

Rajiv: Till grade ten, I studied in Vidya Sagar. For grades eleven and twelve, I moved to Vanavani school, which is a mainstream school. I had a very strange experience while in grade eleven. I was writing my quarterly exams. I used to write with the support of a scribe. But the scribe who came to write for me didn't know any math—he didn't even know how to write; he was that bad! So, what happened was that I got six marks out of two hundred. That was as bad as it could get. The funniest part is that he was doing a PhD in math at the time! That was my first exam in that school.

Dheepakh: Before I was integrated into mainstream school, my parents ran around for two months seeking admission, but drew a blank. Not one school was willing to admit me. I wanted to go to one in particular but the school wasn't courageous enough to take me in because they felt that the other students might bully me.

I finally took a three-hour long entrance test. This was the first time I was writing such a test, one without any breaks. The school was happy with my performance and I was eventually admitted. But first, I was called to the principal's room and he asked me: 'You've written the exam well, but what confidence will you have if you don't have any friends?'

I told her, 'I'll make sure the entire school becomes friends with me.' Exams were always a bit of a challenge, though because of the lack of adequate support.

During my twelfth board accounts exam, I dictated the words 'divided by' to my scribe and she wrote the actual words instead of using the symbol! I lost my temper and asked her what she was doing. She said, 'I'm just writing what you told me to. I don't know anything about accounts.' During another exam, the flying squad came around for an inspection, but they started talking to me and I lost forty-five minutes! I lost thirty-two marks because I couldn't complete the exam. I asked them for extra time but they refused my request.

Srilata: Apart from academics, what were the other challenges you encountered and how did you deal with them?

Dheepak: I actually got the principal to shift my classroom from the second floor to the ground floor. All this happened because of what Rajiv taught me when I was at Vidya Sagar. He taught me not to put up with any injustice. I would also like to recount another experience from my school life. When I was in eleventh grade, a class excursion was planned. The teacher in charge of the planning was concerned about how I would manage. She did not want me to face any difficulty in moving around. She suggested that I talk to the principal. I did so and the principal said, 'If your friends are okay with this, you can go. Otherwise, you can't.' When I conveyed this to my friends, they said, 'If you aren't coming, we aren't going either.' And so, finally, I ended up going on that excursion. I believe in mutual help—my friends helped me out with physical tasks and I helped them in any way I could. At first, my teachers didn't think I was academically strong. This was because they didn't know me too well. But after my first year in school, they realised that I could compete. This is the problem with the mainstream school system: people have to constantly prove themselves.

I faced a lot of problems in my personal life as well. I lost my parents when I was quite young. My dad passed away in 2004. My mom had breast cancer and passed away in 2007. My mom's elder brother decided that I should stay with him, discontinue my education and start working as a clerk in a bank. He did not want me to study. He said I had to take up responsibilities. My school principal had actually offered me a job as a clerk at a bank that was right behind my school compound in West Mambalam. I would have to travel an hour and a half to go from Pallavaram to West Mambalam for that. My three maternal aunts spoke to their brother in my support and insisted that my education continue. I wanted to get a degree. Each of my three degrees have been a struggle. Till 1998, I was in Vidya Sagar; from 1998 until grade twelve, I was a student of Jaigopal Garodia, a school in West Mambalam.

Srilata: What would you say is the role of parents in the lives of persons with disabilities?

Rajiv: Many people with disabilities are not aware of what supports them; they take that for granted. They don't realise that they are being supported at all.

Dheepak: Persons with disabilities rely wholly on their parents for support because they are not aware of their rights. They are made to feel content with that.

Rajiv: Actually, this is a problem, for we all have to get used to new people. But it is not easy to change our support system.

Dheepakh: When we reach a certain point in life, we take our support system for granted and forget it quite easily. Bringing up persons with disabilities is a commitment, one that parents have to make. So, it doesn't work like an achievement they can boast of. But if a person with a disability achieves a small thing like picking up a cup or drinking water from a glass, that is an achievement. The parameters of what an achievement is, differ. You can't use the usual yardsticks to measure what an achievement is when it comes to a person with disability.

Srilata: Would you say that persons with disabilities ought to be given as much exposure to the outside world as possible, so they can develop the skills to cope with life?

Dheepakh: Yes. My parents gave me the utmost exposure. For instance, they used to take me to watch English movies. Till I got to tenth grade, I didn't know Tamil. Exposure is a must for persons with disabilities. My parents were proactive. They taught me using flash cards with alphabets written in large font. I used to watch Wimbledon with my father and was able to recognise Boris Becker. This helped with my school admission. I used to travel by myself when I was in the fifth. Auto drivers would ask me why I was travelling unaccompanied. I would tell them that I was doing this on my own so I that I could manage an independent life after my parents passed away. Because of the way I sit, auto drivers often ask me whether I'm drunk.

Even 'bad' or negative experiences like falling off a cycle are important. I've gotten my head split open by a barbed wire. You can still see the scar. The doctor who administered the tetanus shot asked if I had mental retardation. I shouted at her. She had assumed this was the case because of the way I laugh. When I am in pain, I don't cry.

Rajiv: Dheepak is one of the few who pursued his passion. I was actually interested in astrophysics but because I could not take the science stream in school—I was not allowed to—I could not pursue my passion. Even today, in my free time, I read about astrophysics. And yes, when it comes to commuting by auto, policemen have also asked me the questions that Dheepak is asked. I actually took one of them to task, but not everyone can do it.

Srilata: There are many different ways in which disability is understood and defined. Can you say a little bit about that, especially from the perspective of advocacy?

Rajiv: If you look at the definition of disability as per the United Nations Convention on the Rights of Persons with Disabilities (UNCRPD), it takes into account three factors: persons with impairments, attitudinal barriers and environmental barriers. It is only when an impairment comes into contact with attitudinal and environmental barriers that it becomes a disability. That's why it's called a disability. It's only an impairment, not a medical issue.*

Dheepakh: The way society looks at me makes it a disability. When I go to the airport, my *caretaker*—and not me—will be asked where I'm going. I fought with the airlines when I

---

* The UNCRPD is an international human rights treaty intended to protect the rights and dignity of people with disabilities. The text was adopted by the United Nations General Assembly on 13 December 2006 and opened for signature on 30 March 2007. It came into force on 3 May 2008. The Convention adopts a social model of disability. According to the preamble, the Convention recognises: '... that disability is an evolving concept and that disability results from the interaction between persons with impairments and attitudinal and environmental barriers that hinders their full and effective participation in society on an equal basis with others.'

went to Mumbai. I was denied a wheelchair and lift from the aircraft at the Mumbai airport. I was actually being felicitated in Mumbai but I was forced to sit inside the aircraft for an hour while the other passengers deplaned. And I was literally lifted up and brought down from the aircraft in a way that made me uncomfortable.

I contacted Rajiv and then got in touch with my journalist friend. That's how I managed to get an apology from the airline two days after the incident. The point is, I could do that because I know people, but most people can't. I am not boasting about the fact that I know people. What I am saying is that for others it will be a far worse struggle.

Rajiv: We know how to go about sorting things out and extracting an apology where it is due, but this may not be possible for everyone.

Dheepakh: The reason Rajiv wants to write a book about disability rights is because hardly anyone knows about the subject. Disability is not tied to charity anymore. It is about human rights.

Srilata: Rajiv, what is the nature of your work at Vidya Sagar, at the Disability Legislation Unit?

Rajiv: I worked in different capacities—as a social worker, sharing my experiences with parents of persons with disabilities, and in disability law advocacy with the Disability Legislation Unit.

Srilata: Were you trained in law?

Rajiv: No, not formally. The work I did in terms of advocacy is based entirely on experience. I can tell you about law, especially when it comes to disability rights.

Rajiv: I was a part of the draft committee of Rights of Persons with Disabilities Act (RPDA). This was between the years 2010 and 2013 or so. But then I eventually quit the committee because they didn't accept my views even at face value. My differences with the other members had to do with Section 14 of the act, which was concerned with limited guardianship. I didn't want this section at all. This section enables somebody to decide for you, on your behalf. That's not fair. That was the major contentious point.

Dheepakh: People like Rajiv make their own decisions, but in the case of most persons with disabilities, it is their parents who take decisions. These parents are convinced that their children cannot take proper decisions. What we are trying to say is that persons with disabilities *can* communicate; that they should have the autonomy to take decisions. It is up to us to take the time to listen to them patiently. This holds true even for mental retardation. I've gone through this situation of loss of autonomy myself. I lost my parents at a young age. My dad passed away when I was in the eleventh grade and my mom when I was in second year of college. Then, I had to be looked after by my mom's sister's husband. From then on, every financial decision was his. He believed that I didn't have the experience to take decisions for myself, that I wasn't mature enough. He didn't even care about letting me know what a bank was. I had to go by what he said, could not cross-check what was right or not. This was a mistake on my part too. After I got married, my uncle wasn't happy about my opening a separate account. But I wanted to open one on my own and I did so in HDFC bank. This was important for me. The bank has a ramp and the staff are really flexible and helpful. My uncle used to call my bank to enquire about the bank balance. He did so with all good intentions.

Rajiv: No one will do this to a non-disabled person.

Dheepakh: They were still treating me like a child. Then I told my uncle to stop doing that.

Rajiv: Even now I can't fully operate a bank account. I can't issue cheques because I can't sign.

Srilata: But aren't there other mechanisms such as fingerprints?

Rajiv: Exactly, but banks don't recognise them.

Dheepakh: In his case, he is seen as severely disabled just because of the way he speaks and moves. It's all about perception.

Rajiv: There is a legal aspect too. I'm sure you know about the Contract Act which talks about 'unsoundness of mind'.* But the thing is that there's no definition of unsoundness of mind. It is an outdated act that has been there since 1872. Cerebral palsy is not considered to be a case of 'unsound mind'. But when this condition is present alongside mental retardation, it is considered to be so. The problem is that people tend to judge people with cerebral palsy by physical appearance. So, they conclude that we are incapable of taking our own decisions. In India, most laws are not interpreted properly.

Dheepakh: In most cases, parents feel that their children need to be protected. But only if you allow someone to do something will they learn. You need to jump into water to

---

* A reference to Section 12 of The Indian Contract Act, 1872, which describes what constitutes a sound mind for the purposes of contracting. A person is said to be of sound mind for the purpose of making a contract, if, at the time when he makes it, he is capable of understanding it and of forming a rational judgment as to its effect upon his interests. A person who is usually of unsound mind, but occasionally of sound mind, may make a contract when he is of sound mind. A person who is usually of sound mind, but occasionally of unsound mind, may not make a contract when he is of unsound mind.

learn to swim. Parents will say, 'My child wants to swim.' But they won't let the child jump into the water. In my case I was driven into advocacy. I got to a point when I *had* to defend my rights, my choices. I'm sure Rajiv felt the same. It was when I started associating with Rajiv that I got exposure to disability rights and advocacy. This was back in 2000–01.

Our lives run parallel. We have faced very similar experiences, apart from mine with my relatives.

Rajiv: He has had a tougher time because of his relatives.

Srilata: Tell me about the trajectories that your lives took in your adult years—in terms of college education and work.

Dheepakh: I did my undergraduate in Loyola College and then went to the Asian College of Journalism. I joined *The Hindu* in 2012. When I declared that I wanted to pursue a course in journalism, my uncle said, sarcastically, 'Journalism is for people who have mobility. What can you do on a wheelchair with a course in journalism?' Poonam Natarajan, the founder of Vidya Sagar, spoke to my entire family. She explained to them what my future prospects could be with journalism. But my family remained unconvinced. I had no support at all when I came to write my entrance exam. Somehow, I got through. I passed out of the Asian College of Journalism in 2010–11.

Rajiv: He got a scholarship too.

Dheepakh: Vidya Sagar convinced the college administration to admit me. They said, 'Look, this is a trial. If he comes out with flying colours, it's all well and good. If not, we will try something else.' The college gave me a waiver of 1.5 lakhs. Five years later, my cousin comes to my office with tears in his eyes and tells me that the decision I made that day paid off. I don't like it when other people decide things for me. Who are they to do so? You can't limit anyone's scope. It's not a question of being disabled or 'normal'—it's the same for everyone. How do you know what someone is capable of without giving them an opportunity?

Rajiv: After school, I did a B.Com. from Loyola College.

Dheepakh: He was doing his B.Com. *and* working for Vidya Sagar—both at the same time.

Rajiv: I used to have fourteen-hour days. I worked from six in the morning to eight in the night.

Srilata: Is there something you would like to say about the ways in which you have navigated your personal lives as adults—your marriage, for instance.

Dheepakh: My marriage was a bigger struggle than my education.

Rajiv: Mine, too, was a problem, because both our marriages were love marriages. And both of us chose to marry persons with disabilities. My problem was that no one believed that we could live together without any support. Dheepakh's is a conservative family, so you can imagine. It took around five years for me to get married.

Dheepakh: I was with him all the way through.

Rajiv: That's another thing we've learnt. There's nothing like friendship. No relationship comes anywhere close to a friendship.

Dheepakh: I totally agree. When I was in ninth grade, I figured that friends are thicker than relatives. I met my wife in Thiruvallur, where Rajiv and I were conducting an awareness workshop on legal guardianship. She and I didn't talk to each other, but I liked her instantly. I told Rajiv and my other friends about her, and Rajiv advised me to talk to her. We contacted the organisation and they helped us meet.

Again, my family brought up the question: 'How can two people with disabilities live together?'

I told them, 'If you want me to get married, I'll marry only her.' And then I asked them, 'What would you have done if I had come and stood before you after getting married?' That's when they created a ruckus. Finally, they agreed. But two weeks down the line, they tried to persuade me to postpone the wedding. They cited all sorts of reasons for this. They postponed the wedding by twelve days. That in itself was a bit of a downer for my bride. So, I had to console her. We even considered eloping! That was the toughest part. After we got married, my aunt's husband says he had to convince my family to allow me to marry her. He visited me after I got married and moved to my own house. He asked me why I was not keeping in touch with the family even though they had done so much for me. My wife's mother passed away soon after our marriage. At 1 a.m. in the morning, I was taken to Tiruvallur in a cab by a friend of mine. Following that incident, I bought a car because I wanted one for emergencies. My uncle asked me why I had not even bothered to inform him. My point is—why should I inform him? I have a family of my own. Why should I tell them everything? Do they tell me everything? I have the liberty to make my own decisions.

Rajiv: His wife is from a rural area, so obviously that cultural difference has a role to play too and it is natural for her to be scared.

Dheepakh: I promised her I would not abandon her. My family was looking for wedding halls. I told them we could hold the wedding at Vidya Sagar. They came down to Vidya Sagar, met Poonam, placed the money—Rs 1.5 lakhs—on the table and left. All this, without even speaking to me. From buying dresses to garlands, my friends at Vidya Sagar and I did everything. And we pulled it off. Rajiv, Dhana, Meeenakshi akka and others—everyone came together and helped me. It was a case of friends being thicker than relatives. It was the most beautiful wedding. My wife keeps our house spick and span. Now when my relatives visit, they realise their mistake. They are in touch with her regularly.

Rajiv: But the question is, why should it be harder for us in the first place?

Srilata: What is the relationship like between persons with disabilities and their spouses? Do the latter take on a caregiving role?

Dheepak: Persons with disabilities generally consider their spouses as their caregivers, which is not necessarily the case. And moreover, sometimes these 'caregivers' can also erode our autonomy. Since we are dependent on them, they decide for us—what shirts we should wear, what food we should eat. In case of people with severe disabilities, people do this a lot. There can also be sexual abuse, in the case of men too, and this does not come to light.

Rajiv: It has to do with the person's perspective. Even people who know about disability do this. What I was saying was that your spouse need not always be giving you care.

Srilata: That's not the primary role of a spouse.

Dheepakh: As with every couple, we also have fights. That's how we get to know each other. Then also people look and say 'Oh! They're fighting, they shouldn't have gotten married.'

In most cases, they look for a spouse who can take decisions on behalf of the person with disability. The non-disabled partner tends to become the more dominant one. Without our knowledge, we're going backwards even though we're talking about the human rights model.

Rajiv: It is also easier for men with disabilities to get married than for women.

Dheepakh: A person with disability has to accept reality. If you don't get a non-disabled person as a life partner, you should accept someone with a limited disability who can support you emotionally. The stigma needs to go.

Rajiv: In a marriage, the male partner is supposed to 'protect' the female partner. That becomes an issue for men with disabilities.

Dheepak: People don't perceive us as human beings. They don't recognise our individuality. Some people don't want a disabled person to be in a relationship at all. They think that those of us looking to be in a relationship are dreamers. They attach no value to this desire.

Srilata: There is also a certain discomfort about the sexuality of persons with disabilities.

Dheepakh: That's a taboo which needs to go.

Rajiv: Marriage is not only about sex. That too is something we should realise. It's about a lot of things.

Srilata: Are there other aspects of your lives which have been challenging and which you would like to talk about? How about your living situation—housing, for instance?

Dheepakh: We need support for all sorts of life situations. When I got married, I had no support—financial or emotional. I searched for a house and managed to find one in three months. But Rajiv didn't get a house for three whole years because they don't give houses easily to people with disabilities.

Rajiv: I finally got a house in Perumbakkam, which is 20 kilometres away from Vidya Sagar. It costs me at least Rs 600 each day to commute up and down. I travel for three hours on days when there's traffic and for one and a half hours on good days. When I was looking for a house in Kotturpuram, people asked me questions like, 'How will we go out after setting eyes on someone like you first thing in the morning?'

Dheepakh: People asked me the same question. I would tell them to put themselves in my shoes.

Srilata: Would you say that the most important thing to teach a child with a disability is the ability to talk for himself or herself?

Rajiv and Dheepak (*together and forcefully*): Yes.

Rajiv: But I also disagree with that just a little, because everyone need not be a self-advocate. Some people may just want to enjoy their lives. For example, we have a friend who is clear that he doesn't want to be an activist. Everyone doesn't have to take to advocacy professionally.

Dheepakh: My point is, that he has made a choice but if he finds himself in a situation where he has to fight, he has to become an advocate at that point, either professionally or non-professionally.

Rajiv: Without knowing what your rights are or what your support system is, you cannot advocate.

Dheepak: I was a very quiet person in college. With all these experiences, I have learnt to speak up.

Rajiv: One of my former colleagues at Vidya Sagar told me, 'You were never an advocacy person before but you have learnt to be one now.' The situations that we go through make advocates out of us.

All I Want for Christmas

V.S. Sunder

This piece by V.S. Sunder, retired professor of mathematics at the Institute of Mathematical Sciences, Chennai, is a revised version of an article that first appeared in *The Times of India* on 24 December 2011.

Sunder blogs at https://differentstrokes-vss.blogspot.com/. The blog consists mostly of articles he wrote for *The Times of India* between 2011 and 2012, on issues of access and disability rights. Sunder has been increasingly mobility challenged due to the onset of multiple sclerosis, a neurological condition. He has been actively campaigning for the rights of persons with disabilities and for a more inclusive and accessible society.

Today being Christmas Eve, perhaps I ought to take a cue from children all over the world who prepare their 'I want' lists. In deference to my being a Hindu from Tamil Nadu, however, I suppose my prospective benefactor is not Father Christmas but Tamil Nadu's Amma.* This is consistent with the kindness she has been extending to people with disabilities throughout this month. After all, Amma began by commissioning a fleet of buses equipped with special lifts for wheelchair users, and followed it up with the promise of reserving a three per cent quota for people with disabilities in state government jobs. But before I get around to writing my wish list, let me point you to a few things.

For a start, permit me to highlight some elements of

---

* A reference to Jayalalitha, the then chief minister of Tamil Nadu.

planning, seen even in the latest buildings. These are veritable strokes of genius—that is, if their goal is to ensure that no mobility-challenged person depending on a wheelchair can ever access the buildings in question, or sections thereof. To such a person these buildings are as moats around castles of yore were to hostile bands of marauding invaders.

For a start, a certain number of steps (one, three, five, whatever; any number greater than zero is as effective as any other) must be climbed to get from one level to another. These hurdles in the form of steps manifest themselves in numerous forms. They may lead from the street level to the entrance foyer of the building. In one stroke, they ensure that access to the elevators is denied to anyone who has not climbed the required step(s). An entire section of a room could be at a higher level than others, for instance, when there are split levels, such as in all Japanese houses, where you can (should!) leave your footwear at the lower level before ascending to the clean higher level. They could be the only means to access the roof of a building—even if this building has a hundred floors, and elevators take you all the way to the top floor, you will still have to climb some (ten, fifteen ...?) steps to reach the rooftop with the magnificent view (a popular site for parties!). Auditoria will have enough steps strategically placed that there is no way a person can get to a place from which they can either attend or perform in a play, concert or lecture held there without having negotiated those steps. Prime examples are the Music Academy and the Museum Theatre in Chennai and the J.N. Tata Auditorium in Bengaluru.

I first saw the following stroke of genius in some apartment complexes for faculty at the Tata Institute for Fundamental Research (TIFR) in Mumbai (allegedly a premier scientific research institution in India): the idea here is that if a building has ten floors, elevators only need to halt at five places (at levels 1.5, 3.5 ... 9.5) so you 'only need' to either climb up or down half a flight of stairs after getting out of the elevator to get to the floor of your choice.

One of the most spectacular walkways in TIFR is the one right next to the sea, separated from the water by only a fifty-foot-wide clump of rocks, carefully designed so the waves splash on them furiously and majestically during the monsoon, causing a tremendous spray of water on the walkway. It has been some time since I visited TIFR. It used to be necessary to negotiate many steps before one could get to the walkway. I will be very impressed if some kind soul has arranged for strategically distributed ramps that would permit people like me to again have that uplifting multi-sensorial experience of the sea through sight, feel and smell.

The other thing I have noticed is that dimensions—be it the width of doors, the depth and width of elevators or the width of toilets—are not specified with wheelchair users in mind.

My pessimism has been fuelled by a recent visit to Hiranandani's 'upscale' gated community. My trip was prompted by friends who informed me that I would surely find in this gated community 'a barrier-free and accessible environment in which the quality of my life would be significantly enhanced'. Alas, on going there, I found steps without ramps in most places.

Foremost on my wish list, then, is that agencies such as the Chennai Metropolitan Development Authority (CMDA) be required by law to refuse permissions and sanctions to buildings (at least public ones) which do not satisfy minimal accessibility norms. It is my fond hope that the CMDA will make generous use of the points I have raised above and identify some strict no-no's.

All I want for Christmas is a barrier-free environment!

Coming Out,
Coming Home to Myself

Kim

Kim is a writer, educator and researcher working on disability, governance and identification. They are currently working towards a PhD in education and anthropology. They tremendously enjoy fiction, food and furry pets.

When I first tell my partner I'm disabled, I don't say anything. It is still early in our relationship, and I have been carefully curating how he might perceive my body. I often agree to see him only when I know it is the only thing that I will do that day, hoarding all my spoons* for those few hours. But that day, we begin chatting, him sitting on the bed, me on the floor, and then I can't get up. My knees are locked. My body crumbling. It takes all of my focus and energy to be able to hold my body up and continue with the conversation as if I am not falling apart from the inside. Noticing that we haven't eaten but have done nothing to address it yet, he suggests we go get a meal. Nauseous at the idea of the universe of vulnerability that this will open up, I decline. I'm not hungry; I'd like to continue chatting, I say. But the minutes coagulate into an hour and then there is not much of a choice—our hunger isn't going away (neither is my pain, despite my relentless wishing for it to).

---

* I use the concept of spoons as first explained in Christine Miserandino's piece, 'The Spoon Theory'. Miserandino's piece quantifies energy as spoons to explain how people with chronic illnesses only have a limited amount of energy in a day. The piece was first made available on www.butyoudontlooksick.com.

Although I can still summon and describe the pervasive horror from that moment, my partner barely remembers it. In my head, this formative moment of coming out was nothing quite like I had imagined—mostly because it did not involve any kind of naming or labelling at all. Instead, that day, I asked if he would help me up from the floor, nervously laughing about how both my legs had fallen asleep in the hope that that would turn this hideously embarrassing, endless stretch of time into an intimate moment. He did not laugh with me, nor did he offer an anecdote about how his own legs fall asleep should he sit on the floor. Instead, he suggested that we rest, or that he goes out and gets food. To avoid further humiliation, I gladly took him up on the latter.

Every nervous minute from that time is clearly etched in my mind, although I had no idea then that it would not be the only time when I would have to come out as disabled. Despite having been sick in various ways for quite a while, I did not have the words for what was happening to my body. Not very wisely, I also thought that not having the words, not having a name for the rapid deterioration that my body was going through, would mean that it was not, in fact, deteriorating. Even as I struggled to perform basic tasks that I could previously tackle without a second thought, I didn't think I was disabled. Wrapped tightly in my own ableism and the hesitation emerging from it, I did not think of myself as disabled even when I was unable to leave the bathroom for hours at a time due to what I now know were flares. I was not disabled even when I stopped being able to walk up and down the stairs without pain. I absolutely was not disabled when I began to black out without reason, coming back only to remember nothing.

It was with my current partner that I first started to

come out as disabled. I came out to him and to myself simultaneously. I had previously spent (and do still spend, albeit to a much lesser extent) a considerable amount of each day doing exactly as much as would make me appear able-bodied, often overcompensating for the things I hated about my own loss of physical capacity. Colleagues and friends praised my enthusiasm and energy levels, often expressing amazement at how I was so busy and still able to do it all. I would nod and smile and thank them for their kindness, knowing full well that at the end of many days each week, I would go back home and collapse into bed for hours, often too tired to do basic things like eat or shower. I continued to dig myself deeper into this routine, one that primarily involved running myself into the ground so that I had very little time to think about other things. Among the things I barely registered was that when we moved in together, my partner had begun noticing the things about my disabled body that I had previously thought I was doing a good job of hiding.

None of this noticing, however, was a call out in the ways that I had imagined it would be. It stunned—and often continues to stun—me the ways in which noticing and naming are placed within care work. Reluctant to name the things that I could no longer muster the energy for, like doing my own laundry, I would let clothes pile up until I no longer had anything clean to wear. Without any discussion, my partner began to do the laundry. Noticing what exacerbated my allergic reactions—and knowing that I would not have the energy to clean as regularly as I should have—he began cleaning with a regularity that improved my quality of life, only explicitly speaking about it to ask me whether I felt better after the pillows were vacuumed or the windows were shut. My hard-earned independence and intentional lack of vulnerability had been severely eroded. In the absence of all the accompanying narratives in my head about my own abilities, I had to come home to myself. The self that I came home to was vastly different from the person I had always imagined myself to be. Here was a self that, as I came to learn through years of care work, was nothing to have warranted running away from this whole time.

Even as I accepted care, I struggled with what receiving it meant. I couldn't possibly be sick constantly, often losing multiple days in the week to a constellation of symptoms that I was only slowly starting to collect diagnoses for. And, of course, if I did know what exactly was wrong with me, and was receiving treatment for it, then was it not the case that there was no longer anything that was wrong with me? Half a dozen years into my rotation of debilitating illnesses, a friend (who shared some of my own health conditions) and I were joking about community on Gchat, when they responded, 'Us disabled folks have to stick together.' It felt, at once, like someone had opened a pair of windows in my mind, but also like I was free falling. I turned to my partner, astonished—he was really the only person in the world then who knew both my work and my body. Was I disabled?

This is another moment that he doesn't really remember. He looked up from his laptop, said 'of course' and went back to work. I sat in my astonishment. Did I have a legitimate claim to this category? If I was disabled, now what? Why hadn't he said this to me before? He answered the last one first. He didn't know what the word for it was, but he always knew I was disabled. In the years since then, we have learnt, over and over again, what it means to be disabled. I have picked up more chronic illnesses, taken on less work, taken time off to focus on my health. For the first time in my adult life,

I am not chasing work or school deadlines, left to my own devices to sink into bed for as long as I'd like each day. My capacities shift, my symptoms come together in strange ways and the ableism coursing through my veins comes to mean that I am often not my own best caregiver.

Despite the time off, clearly driven by the premise that rest and focused attention on my health will make it much better than it has ever been, my body is falling apart with a renewed commitment. I withdraw, frustrated, thinking of Atul Gawande's description of the ODTAA syndrome—'One Damn Thing After Another'—deeply bitter that this now applies to my own life. My partner's care work has shifted this time towards a more explicit naming of what is going on with my body. His memory is extensive in this regard, noting what makes me feel better, what makes me feel worse, when I should be more cautious with medication, when I should be going in to see a doctor instead of putting it off. My gastrointestinal issues have increased and we are now especially focused on what I eat, a set of processes that has significant potential to trigger a barely-past eating disorder. It is then that he starts to point out explicitly the disordered consumption patterns that he notices, urging me to bring them up with my therapist.

The strangeness of having only one caregiver does not escape me. When I work up the courage to tell friends little bits about what is happening to my body, they respond with deep empathy, offering care consistently even when I push it away. By now, even though I have long since started to embrace my disabled identity, I cannot find it in me to ask for help in any form. I decline offer after offer—soup, meals, reading material, blankets, company, time with other people's pets, rides to the doctor, referrals to other specialists, logistical assistance, running errands on my behalf. My partner watches, not saying anything, but we start to dance around the question of what it looks like for me to accept other forms of care.

Many years into being sick, I have started to know for myself that the label of disability is not where my lived experiences begin or end. There are circumstances under which I am disabled, and many occasions during which I have to come out as disabled. Unlike many people with more visible disabilities, the question of whether, when and how to identify as disabled comes up in more situations than I would have imagined. With it, too, accumulates a separate kind of fatigue that I had not planned for either—being convinced of my impairments and my abilities, but constantly needing to make clear to other people that I would need accommodations even though they might not think I would need any. I am often terrified and hesitant, but many of these feelings are directed toward new symptoms and the possibility of new diagnoses, rather than toward denying my own feelings and experiences.

As someone who is incredibly social, being on the receiving end of care has allowed me the space to rethink what it might mean to understand independence and community—separately in as much as is possible but also together. My nervousness at being fully known is also occasionally accompanied by the overwhelming relief of being known so deeply. Very slowly, I have opened up to other forms and givers of care, nervous each time that my experiences will not be believed or that acts of care work will be asking too much of the people in my life. I would be lying if I claimed that all care was willingly and generously offered, or indeed that I had not lost more friends than I would like to remember due to my illnesses. For all the truths I write of, I know of many more that influence my own disabled temporality, that I am still working to fully name. Much like the ways in which I imagined that naming my impairments would be a one-time endeavour, not an ongoing process, I know too that my own relationship with receiving care is a process. I continue to be prickly, wary, uncertain and sceptical at the same time as I attempt to be more accepting, patient and generous in spirit, setting myself up for a constant dance between these poles. It feels as though the moments when I come out as disabled are far more often than I could have imagined. At the same time, however, I take comfort in recognising the other side of this coin—the ability I have now acquired to come home to myself.

Vision

Ruth Vanita

Translated from the Hindi 'Nazar' by the author

Ruth Vanita is the author of many books, most recently *The Dharma of Justice in the Sanskrit Epics: Debates on Gender, Varna and Species* (Oxford University Press, 2022). Her first novel, *Memory of Light*, appeared from Penguin in 2020; her collection of poems, *A Hidden Player*, will appear in 2022, and she is now working on a second novel.

I have a terrible headache again today; since morning my head has been throbbing as if someone is hammering away at it on the inside. And that old childhood fear returns—what if I go blind?

'Why do you keep reading all the time then?' Ajay can think of only one reason for my feeling unwell. 'Your eyes are weak—how many times have I told you not to read so much? It's not as if you have to pass any more exams now.'

Exactly what the doctor said to my mother when I was a child. 'Madam, her eyes are very weak. She's in danger of losing her vision. You had better withdraw her from school. Fortunately, she's a girl. No point in her studying too much.'

But my mother didn't agree with him. And the truth is that these days my head aches not only when I read, but a lot of the time. After sending Ajay off to work, I wait for the vegetable seller, then for the cleaning woman, and dispatch all kinds of small and big chores; by evening the ache takes full possession. At night, as soon as Ajay touches me, it speeds up like a train leaving the station. After he goes to sleep, I listen to its steady beat. Perhaps I remain in its embrace even when I'm asleep, because I wake up with a slight pang—the day beginning again.

That is why even though it's hard to get away from all the work at home, I am happy to accompany Shaku di when she goes to volunteer at the Red Cross or a women's association or to interview someone.

Shaku di lives upstairs, with her son and daughter-in-law. She's about fifty years old, cheerful, always ready to chat. I'm the quiet type, so I like the company of talkative people. And Shaku di is not the sort of talkative person who is unaware of anything except the sound of their own voice. Ajay and I often fall out; Shaku di never asks questions or gives advice. She just makes me a cup of tea and talks about all sorts of things to divert me. Not touching the central question, she tries to indicate to me that this knot cannot be untied, so what's the point of struggling with it?

Today, Shaku di is going to a blind girls' home; she wants to write an article on the conditions there, because this is the Year of Disabled Persons. 'The blind boys' home is so big and has so many facilities,' she tells me. 'And here, just imagine, the girls are shut up in small dark rooms like prison cells. The last time I went, the warden wouldn't let me meet the girls. I'll see how she stops me this time.'

A golden afternoon. I am ready on time, but a whole lot of visitors drop in on Shaku di. Finally, after entertaining all of them, she emerges, not having managed to eat any lunch.

'How far is it?'

'Just a ten-minute walk. Near the gurudwara.'

'So, it's right in the centre of the colony, and I didn't even know it existed.'

'You've only been here a year.'

'If you hadn't told me, I probably wouldn't have known even in ten years.'

'Look, it's that house.'

'That one?'

A house like any other; no external sign that instead of one housewife's, many girls' lives are smouldering within.

'Look, what a jail they've made of it.' Shaku di points to the closed windows. 'I've heard they don't let the girls go anywhere. They're not allowed to step out of the gate.'

I begin to feel strangely reluctant as we approach the house. As if we are going to observe some unknown species. What will they think of our arrival? They probably won't like it. I feel quite unfit to talk to them—what am I going there for, with my ignorance and my eyes?

We go in and find the watchman missing. We peek into the office; no one there either. The ground floor is deserted. We can hear girls' voices upstairs.

'Oh, it's 15 August today, so it's a holiday. That's why there is no one here; how amazingly incompetent they are.'

Then I remember; of course, Ajay hasn't gone to office today. He is at a friend's house and will be back early. Shaku di sees her chance. 'Come on, let's go up and talk to the girls. If the warden were here, she might have stopped us.'

We climb the stairs quickly. Three open doors on the first floor. Dark rooms. For a moment we stand there, uncertain. Then Shaku di steps forward. Right next to the door is a bed. There are two other beds in the room too. Four or five girls are in the room, lying and sitting on the beds. On the bed next to the door, two girls lie wrapped in each other's arms, and a soft sound in a monotone, like the rippling of a brook, like a mother's—no, just like my own voice ...

... Jayshree and I used to cycle to college together every

day, racing each other. When the cycles took wing and the sleepy Allahabad morning dazzled awake to the perfume of Jayshree's long hair, her laughter, her intoxicating company, I felt as if she and I would fly like this through life, leaving the world behind, ecstatic at our own pace. Those three years spent with Jayshree now seem like the three hours of a colourful film, from which one emerges into the same whispers in the dark, vulgar hoardings, sharp light and men's sharper stares, but at the time it was no dream. It was waking reality, speaking and laughing. Reality that shook awake with music my half-slumbering heart, opened my eyes to many colours, unwrapped my enfolded desires and set them afloat on the winds.

At that time, I didn't have these thoughts, these words, neither did Jayshree. Just feelings. How many times I wanted to tell her something, something surely very profound, rising up to my throat, and I would say, 'Listen ...'

'Yes?'

'No, it's nothing.' Weeping, that something sank back into me.

My father was transferred and we had to part, still in that same silence. My head on her shoulder, my whole body blossoming, she trembling like a young tree awakened by the breeze, yet we couldn't say anything. As if our tongues had been cut out or we had forgotten our names. Yes, now sometimes words come pouring out.

Not the couple of times I have formally met Jayshree—on those occasions my head feels numb and my body like a chopped-off branch. But in dreams sounds rise to my lips of the kind I'm now hearing. 'Lord knows what nonsense you keep talking in your sleep,' Ajay says. 'I can't understand a word of it.'

Shaku di is asking the girls questions. The oldest girl answers, calmly, but as if on high alert. Emphasising the terrible conditions in which they live, Shaku di keeps asking whether she's longing to go home, and the girl keeps repeating that she is perfectly content living here.

'What work do you do here?'

'We knit mop cloths.'

'How much do you earn?'

'Four annas a cloth.'

'That's all? Don't you want to move to the Rajinder Nagar school where you could study further?'

'No.'

'Why not? Don't you want to study further?'

'No. What's the point of studying?'

Shaku di is speechless. She considers education the only means of women's upliftment. Her father did not let her continue her education and tied a husband around her neck. I too am a bit surprised by this answer. Shaku di tries to expand the girl's horizon; after all, why would such a smart girl want to continue living in this prison?

'But if you study you can advance in the world, you can marry.'

'I don't want to marry.'

Shaku di thinks she is saying this because she thinks no one will marry her. 'Why? Why should you think like that? Just last month Miss Verma who teaches in the Rajinder Nagar school got married. I've interviewed a lot of people there, a lot of men as well. All the men are married.'

'No, I don't want to marry. Absolutely not.'

'But why not?'

'What's the use of marrying?'

Shaku di does not answer this question. Instead, she

begins to talk to another girl. A girl from the hills, smiling, pink-cheeked, playful like a child.

'What about you? You don't want to study?'

'I used to study in the Rajinder Nagar school. I was expelled from there.' She is shy and doesn't speak with the confidence of the older girl.

'Why were you expelled?'

She is silent.

'Shall I talk to them and get you re-admitted there?'

She shakes her head in the negative.

'But why not?'

'No.'

'You don't want to study?'

'Yes, I do want to.'

'Well, then?'

'I'll study here.'

'But there are no teaching arrangements here. You have to study on your own. There you will be properly taught.'

There is no answer, so Shaku di changes the subject. 'What pretty bangles you're wearing. Who gave them to you?'

Her pink complexion turns even more rosy, and she indicates another girl with her head. What love, what pride, what joy on her face ...

Shaku di talks a little more and then stands up to go. And I? Throughout the conversation, I sit silent, tears in my eyes, like a guilty person.

∼

A few days later Shaku di turns up, rather excited.

'Manju, I talked to some women teachers there. They say that all these girls love each other and have formed couples.

That day I felt there was some such thing going on and when I asked, the teachers said clearly, "So what? If they're happy, what is it to you?"'

Gathering all my courage, I manage to say, 'But what is wrong with that?'

'Because they are not allowed to meet boys and they need love and affection, they start embracing and kissing one another from childhood onwards, and as they grow older, they want to live only with women.' She pauses, and then concludes, 'I am going to write about all this in my article.'

So far, I have listened with the wariness of that girl the other day, but now the words come pouring out, not to protect those girls from our insolence, our shamelessness, but as if to protect myself. 'But, Shaku di, if they are happy, why should anyone object? How happily and confidently they spoke that day. They didn't want anyone's pity. They shouldn't be prevented from meeting boys, but how do we know they will be happier with boys? How much happiness and confidence have you and I found with men? How many have found it?'

Shaku di hesitates, then says, 'No, but such things interfere with children's education.'

I feel a gulf opening up between Shaku di and me, which I must leap over. 'But Shaku di, children play these sorts of games with each other in every house. They hide their play, feel afraid and guilty. It's all a matter of how you look at it. We keep repeating what we have been told is right or wrong but the reality may be different.'

'When I talked to the teachers about this they said, "We only care about the exam results, and the pass percentage is 100 per cent."'

'They are happy so why wouldn't it be 100 per cent?

If you write about it who knows how the authorities may punish them?'

'All right, I won't write about this, but the misuse of government funds, the girls not getting proper food and clothing, the low wages, the unnecessary restrictions ...'

'Yes, of course, it's important to write about all that.'

Shaku di has left. I stand by the window. Today, I saw a whole other world just a few steps away from where I live. How much I saw in a few minutes! There are more worlds to be seen—the worlds in me, worlds beyond me, new worlds being made, worlds that could be made. I have to make up for the years, the centuries, I have lived with limited vision.

Delhi, 1983.

I Should Not Ask Random Questions

A Conversation with Gayathri

Twenty-six-year-old Gayathri, on the autism spectrum, is a volunteer at The Lotus Foundation. This conversation has been transcribed here more or less verbatim. The founder-director of The Lotus Foundation, Nandini Santhanam, was present right through and helped facilitate the interaction. Even though it was a bit of a challenge to keep the conversation ball rolling (there was a certain circularity and repetitiveness to it), I found that Gayathri was responsive, eager to be heard, to understand and to be understood.

Srilata: When did you first join Lotus? Tell me how and when this happened?

Gayathri: 2016.

Srilata: How old are you now?

Gayathri: Twenty-six. Married.

Srilata: And what does your husband do?

Gayathri: Manager, HR … Cognizant.

Srilata: And you are volunteering right now at The Lotus Foundation.

Gayathri: Yes. Helping out. Like it.

Srilata: What do you like about being here? Madam[*] was telling me that you worked for a short while in a company?

Gayathri: Internship.

---

[*] Nandini Santhanam, the founder-director of The Lotus Foundation

Srilata: So, you left the company and decided to volunteer here. So, what was it like for you when you were working for that company? Why did you leave?

Gayathri: Because it was too far away.

Srilata: Tell me about the work you do at Lotus?

Gayathri: Gardening. Do you speak Tamil?—I speak Tamil and English.

Srilata: That's great!

Gayathri: I know Hindi. I like Hindi.

Srilata: Do you teach the others at Lotus?

Gayathri: I teach. Yes.

Srilata: Does that make you feel satisfied?

Gayathri: Satisfied.

Srilata: Tell me about your family.

Gayathri: Mother-in-law, father-in law, dogs.

Srilata: Are you fond of them? Are they fond of you?

Gayathri: Fond. Fond of them.

Srilata: When you go home in the evenings, what do you do?

Gayathri: Sleep.

Srilata: How about dinner? Do you cook?

Gayathri: Night. We cook in the night. 7.30.

Srilata: What do you like to cook?

Gayathri: Chapathi, paneer.

Nandini: Don't you go to music class, Gayathri? What sort of music do you learn?

Gayathri: Carnatic music.

Nandini: You also teach Hindi to a child, right? You take tuitions in the evening, don't you?

Gayathri: I take Hindi class.

Srilata: Which school did you go to?

Gayathri: Chettinad Vidyashram, at first. From seventh–Kumararani. Till twelfth.

Srilata: Did you like being in school?

Gayathri: I liked being in school.

Srilata: Both schools?

Gayathri: Kumararani is state board. I didn't like CBSE.

Srilata: Did you have friends?

Gayathri: Lot of friends at Kumararani.

Srilata: What is your favourite subject?

Gayathri: Commerce. Commerce and computer science.

Srilata: Do you have friends at Lotus?

Gayathri: Subashree. She hasn't come today.

Nandini: Subashree is one of our children. She has come back to work with us.

Srilata: Do you watch films?

Gayathri: Tamil movies.

Srilata: Which activity do you like the most at Lotus?

Gayathri: Hindi class.

Srilata: Where did you learn Hindi?

Gayathri: When I was in school.

Srilata: Was it your second language?

Gayathri: Third language.

Nandini (*to Gayathri*): Tell her about gardening, nature walk.

Gayathri: Gardening, nature walk.

Nandini: She likes painting, cooking.

Gayathri: Baking cake!

Nandini (*to Gayathri*): Tell her about weaving.

Gayathri: Weaving.

Srilata: Where do you go for weaving?

Gayathri: WeCan,* Nelangarai.

Srilata: What kind of weaving do you do?

Gayathri: I have woven a lot.

Srilata: Why do you like weaving?

Gayathri: Pattern weaving.

Srilata: What kind of plants do you like to grow in the garden?

Gayathri: Tomato plant, spinach.

Srilata: Is it a vegetable garden?

Gayathri: Vegetable garden.

Srilata: You said you like to bake. Will you bake a cake for me some time?

Gayathri: I will bake one for you some time.

Nandini (*to Gayathri*): Ask her where she works.

Srilata: I work at IIT. I am a teacher.

Nandini (*to Gayathri*): Do *you* want to ask her anything?

Gayathri: Are you married?

Srilata: Yes, I am. I have two children. They are grown up now. My son is in college, my daughter is in high school. She likes music. Do you like music?

Gayathri: I like music …

Gayathri (*to Nandini*): I should not ask random questions, no?

---

* Centre in Chennai for children with autism.

Nandini: Yes, to you it may be meaningful. But to the person you are asking it may not be so. That's why you should not ask random questions.

Gayathri: Wearing yellow today. Day before was my birthday.

Srilata: Belated birthday wishes, Gayathri! And thank you for agreeing to this interview.

BOOK THREE

The Whisper of Your
Head Tilting

Note

What does it mean to see? Is seeing only about sight? Or is there a larger seeing—seeing with the heart, with attentive ears and probing fingers? And what of the things that the sighted do not see?

Getting the Light Just Right

Anannya Dasgupta

Anannya Dasgupta is a poet, art photographer and fiction writer who lives in Chennai. Her short stories can be found in *Mad in Asia Pacific, Queen Mob's Tea House, Out of Print, Aainanagar* and *Bangalore Review,* among other publications. She directs the Centre for Writing and Pedagogy at Krea University, Andhra Pradesh.

'The art of portrait photography is in getting the light in the eyes,' said Javi, adjusting the umbrellas to light my friend Kashif's face, who was patiently allowing himself to be a subject as I got my first lessons in setting up basic studio lighting. *Light in the eyes*—that was what stuck in my head as I began teaching myself to photograph people after years of resisting exactly that.

'Why the sudden interest in people?' asked Javi, an Argentinian postdoc in a biology lab, who also ran the photography club at the university's recreation centre and knew well of my reluctance. I had cornered him over a cup of coffee and begged him to help me out. Having recently moved out of campus housing to a rented studio apartment in Highland Park, I was hard up.

'Rocks, buildings and trees don't care to be photographed and certainly don't offer money for prints,' I said. Plus, as Javi knew well enough, as a foreign student, the only extra money to be made was from low-paying, hard-to-come-by campus work-studies. Studio portraits were expensive and I had a feeling that folks on campus who wanted a decent mugshot wouldn't mind paying a little cash if I did a good-looking-enough job. Javi had agreed to show me the ropes; he had lent me the gear I would need to practice on my own, and in return, had requested me to help him out with a photography event he was organising in the neighbourhood as a part of its Christmas celebrations.

'We are offering to do studio portraits for free for two days. We will set up at the Reformed Church on Second and Magnolia. I am getting some photographers together. You have three weeks to get good at this—' The last bit trailed behind him as he got up and left. I could feel his eyes twinkling, while mine darkened with worry.

The light in the eyes, I have to get the light in the eyes, I repeated in my head as I met the challenges of portrait photography in my makeshift studio, extending from my dining area to the tiny kitchen, and cajoled and bribed friends to be practice subjects. I saw faces clam shut in front of the camera, saw people stubbornly retreat behind their photo faces and, as I learnt to draw them out by getting them to talk about what they cared about, I realised Javi was right. When my subjects returned to their faces, in spite of the camera, and were fully with me again, their eyes lit up. All the paraphernalia of lights and carefully placed reflective surfaces that I had set up to be just right were meant to catch the light in the eyes. The light I was after was *in* the eyes. As my body absorbed the mechanics of the camera and the setup of lights, I focused on the small pinprick of white that would appear in the pupils. With it came the crevices that started at the corners of the eyes and ran across the face to make a smile grander than the Grand Canyon. I learnt to let the face compose itself around the eyes. My picky human subjects started to make appreciative noises about their portraits but the definitive sign that I was ready for the photography event came from Javi himself. He responded to one batch of photos I had emailed not with his usual summary of everything I had got wrong with the aperture or the distance, not even with the dreaded lecture on the offending shadows on the wall behind or, worse, on the face, but with a single emoji of a winking smiley.

On the big day, I stood in trepidation outside the door of the Reformed Church, despite the smell of cinnamon and coffee that wafted out every time someone pushed open the door. I had moved from campus housing to this neighbourhood because I was tired of living in a student dorm in the middle of what felt like an interminable parking lot. I wanted to be in a community of real people of all ages, doing real people things. But I had not quite understood what community living meant in that moment in post 9/11 suburban America. I was constantly aware of being outside whatever made up the heart of this place. I was transient; I didn't belong. But there is only so long one can stand outside in the week-before-Christmas cold in New Jersey, so I went in with my trepidation, not quite expecting to be swept into the day without a moment to think.

We were full up, all five photographers that Javi had lined up for the two days. That no one, not even the other photographers, could tell that I was only three weeks into the game had me feeling very satisfied and even somewhat smug. My unbelonging momentarily forgotten, I was blissfully unprepared for what was to happen the next day.

I had spent the first part of the morning photographing several theatre students who made it really easy to find their face in the photos as I tracked their pupils for the right moment to hit the shutter. As I was finishing up, I noticed a young woman walk in and sit down on the chair meant for the person next in the queue. A dog dutifully flopped on the floor next to her feet as she folded the cane looped on her wrist and held it in her lap.

Sensing the last person leave and my footsteps approach, she stood up, holding out her hand to shake. 'Hi, I'm Meagan and this is Spot, my guide dog.' She told me that she was new to the neighbourhood and had moved for a part-time job at the library. 'I am also a writer,' she said. 'I need some photographs for a website I am getting done to publicise my just-out novel.' Her eyelids fluttered, barely open, her neck swayed from side-to-side and there was a big smile on her face. I shook her hand and introduced myself, saying the customary nice-to-meet-yous, as I felt a hollow in my gut for the obvious inadequacy of the technique I had spent the last few weeks perfecting. *How was I going to do this?* Panic rose in my throat, drowning the words that were supposed to come next. 'Umm ... you'll have to lead me to where you need me to stand for the pictures.' Megan made up for my silence, possibly aware of and not new to the awkwardness of such encounters.

I led her to stand four feet from the backdrop, Javi's injunction against backdrop shadow somehow heightened in my mind as I adjusted the light stands to her height. 'What's your novel about Megan?' I started on the preliminary banter meant to keep people from retreating from the camera. As Megan described her novel, I noticed that she wasn't shy of the camera at all; it didn't matter that it was there. The animation on her face, though, grew as I asked her for more details of her book and probed her on the plot. The only problem was I didn't know how to compose her face to retell its liveliness. My photos worked because the faces looked back at the viewer in a direct, stirring gaze. I scanned her face in the viewfinder, grasping at straws, unable to replace in my head my organising formula of composition. The nose, the mouth—the other candidates on a face—seemed not to yield what the eyes had. In that moment, my world separated into subjects I had learnt to see and those that I had not. As a photographer, I could not show what I didn't see.

Javi had taught me well enough that I turned out a good-enough picture of Megan. I settled on a profile shot—head bent forward, long hair falling on one side of the face and tucked behind the ear on the side facing the camera, eyelids lowered, mouth closed but smiling—as I complimented her on her book. I made the photograph black and white.

I heard from Megan a few days after I had emailed her the photo; her website designer loved her author portrait. But it bothered me. It bothered me that in the photograph I took, it was not possible to tell if the person was sighted or blind.

~

With the word-of-mouth advantage that the free portrait event gave me, my dalliance with portrait photography grew serious and got me enough extra cash to pay my rent comfortably and even invest in my own gear as I reluctantly parted with Javi's. Between my research, teaching, the photo gigs and a summer trip home to Delhi, I hadn't gone for my neighbourhood photo walks, which is probably why I missed running into Megan sooner. When I did, it turned out that she lived only one street over from me. We ran into each other at the check-out line at the grocery store. We started chatting and ended up at the coffee shop to talk some more. We chatted about her work setting up the Braille section in the library, my research, her family of older siblings in South Jersey, my family in India, my recent trip to Delhi, her partner Mark, who was also legally blind and finally about her pregnancy, which was making her family anxious and sceptical in equal measure. The evening ended with the first of many invitations to each other's homes.

Not long after that, I made my way to Megan and Mark's house with a special present. I had a photograph of the Jama Masjid from my Delhi trip etched on a thin sheet of metal and put in a frame without the glass, all courtesy of a friend in the art department. The domes, arches, minarets and the central hauz* stood out in relief, as did a scattering of pigeons in the sky. Eyes shut, I ran my fingertips along the etching, uneasily sensing my way through a familiar image cast onto an unfamiliar terrain. It was still light I when walked up the stairs to the second-floor apartment where Megan and Mark lived. They welcomed me in and by the time we finished catching up on the Jama Masjid and the Delhi of the Mughals, it was dark; it was also time for the promised cup of tea. Megan got busy getting tea ready. Mark started filling up bowls with nachos and dips, both of them laughing and chatting per usual. Me? I sat where I was, in the dark, unable to see well enough to go and help, and too embarrassed to say out loud that I couldn't see. The blinds were drawn and not even the ambient street light made it in, the only light a blue glow from the gas stove that was bringing the kettle to a boil. Finally, it was Mark who took note and asked, 'Hey, do we have the lights on, can you see? She'd need the lights, wouldn't she?' We all burst into laughter as the lights were switched on to fix the disability of the sighted guest.

---

* Water tank in Urdu

In a few months, little Hugh was born, and I became a part of the family as a godparent. Over the next two years, Megan, Mark, Hugh and I bonded on the edges of a neighbourhood that seemed to cluster on familiarity. There were rich White folks from the banks of the Raritan up to Fourth Avenue on the north side, different denominations of Jewish folks and their temples, mostly on the south side up to Second, the Korean Methodists and other affluent East and South Asians up to the Fifth Avenue and then, from the Sixth onwards, an assortment of working class Black, Brown, White, Latino, and graduate students like me made up this neighbourhood of differentiated familiars all the way up to the edge of the next town. It was good to have finally found my bearing and my sense for people who, at least in all appearance, belonged to each other. In that, I was fortunate to not have only the community of foreign graduate students to relate to. I would happily babysit Hugh on days Mark was away and Megan needed to get some writing done at home. If I could mind the baby, she could still take breaks to feed him and get some more or less unbroken mental time for writing. I ended up spending time with Megan and Hugh in the ordinariness of days of caring that make women into mothers and aunts. Whatever self-doubt may have wracked Megan at other times, to see her feed or change Hugh made me feel like I was all elbows in comparison. On days such as those, being on life's periphery and on the neighbourhood's margin had no bearing on this little centre of the universe.

In the meanwhile, my portrait photography brought all kinds of people from campus and the neighbourhood to my kitchen studio as I learnt that good photographs were rarely made by following rules. When I could take the liberty, I photographed people outdoors. I'd ask them to bring a friend along so they could chat and forget about me doing my thing with the camera. I had begun to let my camera become an extension of my shoulders, my hands, my feet, all parts of my body that I pressed into service, as much as I did my eyes.

Before long, my graduate programme came to an end; I submitted and defended my PhD and decided to move back to India. But before I did, I knew I had one thing to do that I had wondered how I would do differently now, after all these years.

I asked Megan if I could do a family portrait.

Early autumn evenings in New Jersey are the time of magic light. We met in the park by the riverbank. Hugh saw me from a distance, freed himself from his father's grip and ran towards me, Spot bounding protectively behind him. Our usual outdoor greeting was for me to hold him by his arms and spin him around till he squealed to be let go, only to pester me to do it again. By the time Megan and Mark caught up with us, Hugh was a heap of giggling mess on the grass, being licked by Spot.

'Where do you want us for the pictures?' Megan asked.

'Right where you are is good,' I said.

Mark picked up Hugh, brushing grass off his clothes. 'Is his face grubby?' he asked, handing me a tissue. I wiped Hugh's face and got ready to photograph this family of three that I had come to love as my own.

Among the many photos I took that day, my favourite photograph, the one that hangs printed and framed in my study at home in Delhi now, is the one in which the three of them are enveloped in a soft bokeh of yellow-and-orange light from the fall leaves on the trees. Megan's face is turned up, laughing. Curly-haired Hugh has his arms around his father's neck, his head turned around to look thoughtfully at something past the camera. Mark, never to be seen without his dark glasses, has his face towards Megan, saying the thing he was saying that was making Megan laugh. None of them are looking at the camera. Light is pouring out of every pixel in that photograph. For once, I had managed to make the camera disappear to draw the viewer into the intimacy and joy of this family portrait of two blind parents and their sighted toddler. People tell me they get goosebumps seeing this picture; in making it, I had finally got the light just right.

Touched by Magic

Nachiket Kelkar

Dr Nachiket Kelkar is an ecologist who studies freshwater biodiversity, Ganges river dolphins, fisheries-dependent human livelihoods and socio-ecological change in the Gangetic river-floodplains of Bihar. At present, he heads the Riverine Ecosystems and Livelihoods programme at the Wildlife Conservation Trust, India.

It was still dark when Nisha awoke. Her grandmother stirred and grumbled, telling her to go back to sleep. For Nisha, darkness was a constant companion. That day she did not want to sleep more. She sat up on her creaky bed, folded her slightly dew-dampened blanket and reached out for the tumbler of water on the wooden stool beside her younger sister's pillow. It was as if her fingers had eyes: tingling with the sensation of knowing that her thirst was about to be quenched, they firmly retrieved it. If the tumbler fell and woke everyone, it would certainly invite her grandmother's fierce cursing. After drinking, she made her way down the creaky wooden stairs of her home and sat down on the cold porch. The gentle and warm westerly breeze woke up her skin like an anticipation of something special. Her father, Bhagatram, would be returning after fishing the whole night in the river. Nisha could not see, but she knew that by the time her father returned the sky would have turned a faint lilac or mauve or pink, for it would be dawn. Her memory of this dawn sky was from eight distant years ago, when she was just six years old. When she had turned seven, her eyesight had faded away irreversibly, which the doctor said was due to chronic malnutrition. Her mother had passed away soon after, and Nisha, at fourteen, took care of her sister, Chanda, and two even younger brothers, Jugnu and Sonu. Their names meant 'silver moon', 'firefly' and 'golden'—and they could all see with their eyes. Nisha's name meant 'the night' and she could see too, but only with her hands, ears and the pores of her skin.

One of her daily chores was to get her siblings ready for school. She had had to leave school after she lost her eyesight. But she had taught herself several things even then—through a combination of what she could remember of things and what her friends and siblings told her and what she touched, smelt, tasted and felt. When their father came back with his catch, she and Chanda would help him sort the fish. Nisha was the expert of the two in knowing which type of fish had been landed. Chanda would complain, 'All fish look grey and silver,' but Nisha could discern all of them by touch. The boari with its big whiskers, the aria with its flat snout, the patasi with its soft but spiky shoulder-spine and the darhi with its peculiar scales and depressed nostrils. The fish also carried the distinctive scents of where they were caught—in the main river, or in the side-channel inlet, or in a deep pool of the Ganga.

That morning, Bhagatram did not return alone. There were three other fishermen with him, all muttering under their breaths, as they worked to haul up a huge fish on the ghat by the river. A crowd had gathered around to see, Nisha understood from the commotion. The fish, weighing nearly 120 kilograms, was brought to their house and placed on the porch. Soon, the excited chatter arose of everyone waking up and crowding to see what the matter was. For once, Nisha did not know what fish this was. 'It is not a fish, Didi, it is the soons,' Chanda cried out, as Jugnu and Sonu also ran out to see. Nisha had heard of this river animal, which people said gave birth to their young and fed them its own milk, and had magical powers. But she had never experienced it from so close. She ran her hands over the dead creature's body—it was cold, smooth and scaleless, and had a long beak with very sharp teeth. Enormous, it had begun to give off a horrid stench. Her index finger landed on a tiny pore near its beak, which her sister said was its eye. The eye was really tiny, like a shrunk buttonhole. Bhagatram and the other fishermen conferred in hushed voices about what to do. The dead river dolphin caught accidentally in their net was an endangered animal and if the authorities caught a whiff of it, they would all be fined, or their nets confiscated. With such a penalty they wouldn't be able to fish for maybe a fortnight, and that would further stress their meagre incomes.

'Maybe we could chop it to pieces near the riverside garbage dump and use the oil,' one suggested, but the other two thought it would be best to tie it down with large stones and drown it before anyone from the city saw it. They tied stones around its flank and pushed it into the river. The westerly breeze picked up and blew eerie and sad into the villagers' households as the soons was returned to the river.

Chanda hugged Nisha tightly, tears rolling down her cheeks. Nisha also felt a lump in her throat—but overcame it, as she consoled Chanda. But it was not just sadness that Nisha felt; she didn't have the words for what she was feeling. When she had run her hands over the cool skin of the dead soons, felt its small button-eyes on her finger-tips, she had become somehow connected to it. In the following days, as the village all but forgot about the soons, Nisha grew maddeningly curious about it. Whoever she asked would tell her that this animal was magical, but the harried adults around her had little time to answer her questions. She even picked up the courage to ask her father one day, after his return early morning, if she could go along with him on his boat so she could hear a soons breathing, alive in the water. Secretly, she thought that being close to a live soons might help her divine its magic. Her father was reluctant and only half-heard her request, saying, 'A didi from the city will come to meet me in the afternoon. Wake me up when she comes.' Then he disappeared inside the house to rest after another long and tiring night that had yielded very little catch. Nisha's spirits dropped, as she now saw no other avenue to learn about the soons that had taken to haunting her asleep and awake. She went about her day so despondently that even her grandmother let her off her kitchen duties. Nisha sat on the corner of the porch, brooding and thinking of the soons, waiting for her siblings to return home from school.

'Is this Bhagatram's house?' A voice trailed into Nisha's ears and startled her out of her reverie. She raised her head in the direction of the voice. 'Are you the didi from the city?' The soft voice broke into warm laughter, and replied, 'Yes, I suppose I am. My name is Asha. Is Bhagatram-ji your father? Is he home?' Nisha scrambled to her feet, feeling this stranger's attentive gaze on her.

'Yes,' she replied, growing suddenly awkward. 'Please sit, I will call him,' she said and ran inside. Having woken up her father, she carried a tumbler of water for the visitor, handed it to her and retreated behind the door. She hung on to every word that was exchanged between this didi and her father, her ears catching fire at the repeated mention of a single word: soons.

As Nisha's luck would have it, Asha didi was a biologist studying the soons, or the Ganges river dolphin, and needed a boat to take her mid-river every day for a few hours for the next week that she planned to live in the village and conduct her research. Bhagatram had readily agreed, for this would supplement his meagre income. Unlike the harried adults around her, Asha didi always seemed to have time for Nisha's questions and had more answers about the soons than anyone else she knew. Chanda told Nisha that Asha didi carried a funny looking device in her hands, wore wires that led to something in her ears and was always writing furiously in her notebook, especially as she talked to the fishermen. Asha didi took to coming by the porch in the late morning, when the children had gone to school and Nisha would be doing some chore her grandmother had set her to. In no time at all, Nisha had described the dead soons, plied Asha didi with all her burning questions and expressed her wish to be on the boat to experience the magic of the soons. Asha didi happily shared stories on the life of this riverine mammal, its special feeding habits and why its numbers were declining. She also told Nisha why it was called the soons: 'For its deep breathing sound when it surfaces above the water.'

Nisha had asked her a few times 'What makes them magical, Asha didi?' but never got an answer. But Asha really wanted Nisha to have her wish. She had grown fond of her and wanted to do something special for her. On a Sunday, Asha rounded up all the children of the house, paid Bhagatram extra and asked him to take them all on a river expedition, to a place where she knew the soons would gather to feed. This was the first time Nisha was to be on their boat and on the river. She had been so near the river and the sound of its water and the smell of its banks, but never been on it. She whispered to Asha didi that she was tingling with excitement for what they were about to see. She wanted to hear the soons breathe. Then, growing thoughtful, she said, 'For such a large mammal, they have really tiny eyes, Asha didi. I have touched them. They were like small buttons.'

Asha lay her arm around Nisha and drew her close, 'You know, Nisha, the soons does not need eyes. Its eyes are so tiny because its river world is so dark. But it knows all that is going on by sound—except for these tiny nets that fishermen use, which it can't detect and gets caught in. Remember I told you that the soons emits sounds that help it figure out the shape and texture of fish and other objects in its way? Soons calves detect thin electric signals of fish and catch them—like how your fingers tingle when they tell apart different fish. They also swim close to the river bottom and brush their flippers on the floor. As they can't see, they need to understand their surroundings through touch.'

Asha didi's words fell on Nisha's ears and skin like raindrops on parched earth. She felt herself becoming so light that she might even have flown away; she felt the magic of the soons, a magic she shared with them. Like her, they, too, did not need eyes to see. Soons! There was a loud splash near the boat, a thorough exhalation from a soons that had just surfaced and a few drops splashed on Nisha's face.

'Here they come!' Asha didi cried out. Chanda, Jugnu and Sonu whooped in delight, but Nisha sat still, her heart too full to move. Asha plugged a pair of rubber wires into Nisha's ears. 'Listen.' A series of clicks, creaks, crackles and bursts filtered into her ears. Nisha listened intently. They appeared like meaningless sounds to everyone else on the boat, but they were words that the soons spoke, only to her—in an unknown language that had touched her by magic.

As Though a Tidal River

Geeta Patel

A professor at the University of Virginia, Geeta Patel began her intellectual life as a science geek child, whose world was made possible by hosts of beings. Her avid curiosity led her to several degrees in interdisciplinary sciences combined with philosophy, leavened by varied perspectives on South Asia. She has written two academic books and edited three special issues of journals, that mingle poetry, politics, law, theory, science, media, colonialism, nations and states, sexuality, policy, loss of the tongue, political economy and financialisation. The lockdown led her, rather unexpectedly, to fashioning her own lyric.

It's the sort of thing one doesn't even notice until one is graced with the reprieve of a small pause. Rather like a tidal river abating, the past shows itself as the silt that alerts one to the water's steady retreat. And what I noticed was this—my world had blurred out. Everything I looked at, sensed, felt was through a haze, that is, if I even realised there was something there, beyond me. But even more acute was the realisation that I, my thoughts, the verges of skin, muscles taut, sharp pincer grieving, the startle of joy: all were muddy; almost nothing there to sense with all my fingers. And I could not, however much I tried to, bring them into focus. It was as though I had disassociated from my entire sensory being and so lost the world I inhabited. And I clearly needed someone or something to help me see through to what was transpiring.

All this happened during an odd time in my life. I was a graduate student at Columbia University, living with a peculiar queer couple. One rather lovely room, big windows, a bed, a desk that had once been someone's dressing table, perhaps with them perched in front of a mirror, or so I had envisioned when I bought it—a lady table. Though I was no lady. I had very few resources and what I did have needed to be conserved quietly, and some of it stowed away beyond my two meals for a treat. Occasional forays into the kitchen with special permission. I think of that kitchen now as the Noida–Delhi border, ijaazat* messaged on a phone so I could breach or trespass into it.

This was an odd time, when I was also tussling with a body that seemed to be falling to bits. Looking back, I see now that I had embarked on a journey into disability, but then it just felt as though various pieces had stopped working as they once had. My legs had given way after years of pounding them down, running marathons in Keds. My knees had turned into ostrich eggs, the skin stretched almost to the point of tearing, so that I had to lift my calves off my bed and gently settle my feet into standing, cane waiting for the extra support it offered.

I called myself a cripple, in that tenderly ironic humorous way people who are acutely disabled have, grimacing in laughter with my orthopaedist at the time. Perhaps because I had to be so painstaking about every motion, every step, is why I didn't notice what had happened to my hearing, seeing, touching. When I saw my withdrawal, if seeing is what one can call it, I thought of it as so deep a secession of my heart that it could not be found.

In retrospect, I have begun to notice how many people around me are as I was at that time. But for the me then,

---

* Urdu for permission

it presented a strange burden. I had grown up in a violent household that is almost beyond description, for violence can be that way, where words fail. And in that flat, by the sea, only my nani and I were willing to look at it for what it was. To bear it, because that was all a child could do. My nani taught me how to hone down, to sense the sifting of wind, to fall willy-nilly into wave froth ebbing, to hover over tide pools and whisper to crabs and the sliver flash of fish, to hear every rise and drop of bird sounds. In other words, to meditate so that pauses stretched their arms out into the languor of the infinite. Here lay my repose, my reason for holding onto life. So, when it was lost to me, or I slowly opened myself up to its not quite being there, it felt as though the small hope that kept me afloat had been whisked away—by me. I knew I had to find a therapist, but I had only the occasional dollar tucked into a sock I kept for such times. When I first went looking, I assumed that a therapist's work lay in listening to me, while she sat there silent on her chair, asking questions to help me along the path to healing. Little did I know that it was in the relationship, the back and forth, the interfaces that something unexpectedly transformative was shaped.

After much scouring, I happened upon the Institute for Contemporary Psychotherapy that let me pay ten dollars a session. And I was given a therapist—Adrienne Asch,* who was working on her PhD. I meandered slowly to our first

---

* Asch was a pioneer in disability studies and the feminist interrogations of bioethics, among many other things. She died of cancer that recurred in 2013. *Women with Disabilities: Essays in Psychology, Culture, and Politics*, published in 1987, was one of her books. I spent ten years with her at Wellesley College, where we both taught, eons after our initial foray into therapy. For more details, look up Sara Bergstresser's piece at http://www.voicesinbioethics.net/features/2014/03/12/adrienne-asch.

session at her office, my hand reaching for trees I couldn't quite discern to augment my cane. I entered her office. She was sitting there, slender white cane leaning against her chair, and her eyes so paled out, lids softly closed; she was blind. The only thing that came out from me was an apology—I told her I would have to constantly be in arrears; ten dollars was more than I could manage. It meant that I would have to convert meals into nibbles on biscuits. She laughed and, in that quick bark she had, said, 'Doesn't matter. Why have you come?' And nothing came out, nothing, no words fell into my head, no words against my breath, nothing pushing against my tongue. Session after each ten-dollar session. Nothing. I knew that it was not Adrienne, something about the ordering of the room, the desk, the chair, the therapist, me on another chair was askew. And that pause became interminable.

So, I began to read whatever I could scrounge or happen upon about psychoanalysis in India. This was the early 1980s, when that history had not been written so copiously about, let alone known easily. Girindrashekhar Bose[*] suggested routes to South Asian psyches but, though curiosity provoking, they had no clues to my conundrum. I finally encountered a short piece by Sudhir Kakar[†]—and it threw something open. In my next session, I told Adrienne about it. What Kakar had noticed (and this is my paraphrase from that time) was that when he held therapy sessions in the confines of his office, patients

---

[*] Girindrasekhar Bose (1887–1953) was an early twentieth-century South Asian psychoanalyst, the first president of the Indian Psychoanalytic Society. He carried on a twenty-year dialogue with Sigmund Freud. Bose's doctoral thesis, *Concept of Repression* (1921), blended Hindu thought with Freudian concepts.

[†] Indian psychoanalyst, novelist and scholar who has worked in the fields of cultural psychology and the psychology of religion.

fidgeted, wiggled their gaze around the room, dribbled out trivial pointers about its various features. Unexpectedly, one time he had to hold a session in the living room, children frittering in and out, calls that floated in from the street, the same patient burst into uncontrolled volubility. Adrienne and I came to an agreement. We would try out sessions in her living room. It had to be early in the morning. She would make coffee and breakfast. I would help her pick her clothes after and walk with her—our pace was in tandem—to the subway entrance.

Everything changed. I won't say that I was exactly Kakar's patient. It was still painstaking business, words winnowed out sometimes so slowly that it felt as though the basket weave had been clogged and rice would not give up its husk. But words came; however it happened, they came. I think that entering Adrienne's life, the door that opened into a small space, the chair I tucked into facing a window, the kitchen a mere sliver on my left, offered me a kind of solace and trust that broke open my habitual turtle-duck-its-head-back-into-heavy-brown-checked-comfort-shell mode. But it was something else as well.

I think that when you are sighted there is one really important thing that evades your notice because you aren't attuned to knowing that you do it all the time. And that is this: we hide in plain sight. I mean that we become masters—kalaakaars*—of visual dodging, fudging, hedging. Our grammar, our choreography of all the pretences we have, are cued into our body to be seen, and as it is seen. And so, we get away with them. I was having one of those moments of hiding—except, of course, as is the case with hiding, I didn't

---

* Hindi for performer/artiste

know I had concealed something, ferreted it away and was playing out a con game with myself visually. I might as well have been Kakar's patient in his office, in that I made what was an inane observation on myself, and I thought I was being so clever. I don't even remember what it may have been, I just remember its framing.

Adrienne ducked her head and said, 'Why are you so uncomfortable?' And what flashed for me was, 'How the eff did she know that.' And session after session, it was as though Adrienne could literally 'peer' through the fold in my shoulder, turn the skin in my fingers x-ray translucent to the bone. It was utterly unnerving. I was constantly flummoxed—when I held something in abeyance, held something back, practised some sort of evasive manoeuvre that would detour me away from what I needed to 'see', Adrienne caught it up in the net of her quiet questions. I finally brought it up with her and she turned to face me, and said, 'All the clues are in your each shift on the chair, the way your fingers sound when they clench, the whisper of your head tilting.' Puzzling over what she said alerted me to my visual iconographies of deception. And Adrienne began asking me to describe with voluminous finesse what she had noted. What I didn't realise until it began its snail shift was that slowly, so slowly, as I gave myself over to language that spoke me, the world came back to me. The tree outside the window wafted into sight, green sprightliness, the fluff of pink as flowers budded, the abrupt acid of the coffee Adrienne preferred, the sharp tang of piss as I walked haltingly beside her to the subway. The feeling of the beads that we picked for her to wear that morning, their soft wood warping slightly in the heat of that summer. And I began to painstakingly open the Godrej locked closet of memories. One turn of the key at any one session.

My parents decided to 'visit' New York that summer. And I knew that as terror gnawed away at my sinews, I would lose my senses again. Adrienne surprised me by suggesting that I numb myself on Valium, float across crowded New York streets in a haze. I knew Adrienne did not exactly approve of medicinal aids or abettors. So, I asked her why she would want me to resort to them, use them to do what my psyche would have done anyway. And the question led us to delve into what had drawn me so deep down that I was lost to myself. What we talked about was that disassociation, the process that had got me to seek her out, was really my psyche's medicine cupboard. It had kept me from hurtling into another sort of oblivion. Now that I had been working through it with Adrienne's help, the dissociation had weakened. My psyche no longer had access to its medicine. But it was okay to have access to it on my terms, when I needed it. I had to learn, Adrienne said, in the keenly still way she sometimes had, to parse the quiet edges of my being as it careened into numbness, trail it the way I would were I to follow a red ant across smoothed-down floor. Coax it. So that I could gently lure my senses back into belonging to me again. But sometimes nothingness was a gift given to hold the horror in its place. To send dread back to the there in my spirit, its place in my past. Now was now, and my sporadic blindness my help, the stick that I could tuck under my shoulder, my erstwhile cure, my repose. And when I was done with it, my blindness would still be waiting for me in its unobtrusive tranquil corner.

My legs have continued to falter when I least expect them to, and along with an entire stable of walking sticks and crutches that hold my body up, I have this buttress as well—each available to me because I painstakingly learnt what they were and how I could avail of them.

The Art of Description: A Blindness Perspective

Hemachandran Karah

Dr Hemachandran Karah teaches English literature at IIT Madras. He is interested in researching on themes such as disability, health, the language question, literary criticism and musicology. The hallmark of humanities scholarship lies in its rare capacity to enrich responsible world-views, empathy, justice and care. Karah's activism as a teacher and a scholar caters to such a goal. In addition to academic writing, Karah regularly contributes to newspapers and magazines.

Without the art of description, one cannot access anything, not even personal experiences. The ability to describe is truth, power, knowledge and much more. That's why we should cultivate this art across learning environments. It is known to serve diverse communities organically. Blind people, for example, rely on the art of description to live, learn and flourish amidst ever-changing visual realities. Living and learning are also political manoeuvres. An exposure to what constitutes political manoeuvring is as priceless as the art itself. How about a flashback to my blind school? We will begin there, and learn a thing or two about blindness and the subtle art of description.

'Do you know how a sparrow looks?' Sister Florence tapped me on my shoulder. Kumar and I squeaked. Sister Florence was our blind school teacher. That day she smelt a rose. 'Did you steal that rose from the church garden?' A mild thud landed on my back. 'Shush, show me your hand.'

Sister Florence began drawing an image on my palm with a pencil. I quickly yanked it away. 'Sister, it is tickling me!' 'Okay, Okay, I will be careful this time, darling.' She pulled my palm again, this time drawing the image of a sparrow with her index finger. 'This is the beak,' she began artfully. I must say that the beak was as pointed as our Taylor frame type.* Little square ... some zig-zags ... and at last the tail ... it must have been as long as my pinky!

Whenever we heard sparrows fly by, they sort of left an image of them in our palms. Aeroplanes, ducks, Mount Everest, elephants and all the rest made their way into our palms this way. In a way, it is Sister Florence's art of description, and not arbitrary words per se, that helped us children gradually master our environments.

As I recall this anecdote, I cannot help but reaffirm the idea that the art of description, of teaching description, is akin to mothering. It makes available realities that can nourish someone from within. We chew, swallow, digest and enliven words that come with contexts and descriptions. Without mothering and without careful description, inner enrichment becomes almost impossible. In fact, words, concepts, notions, and the rest may remain inside us as undigested foreign objects. With undigested foreign objects piling up gradually from the inside, all of us may grow up to become polished data banks, and nothing more.

Even as the art of description is akin to mothering, it can, in some instances, begin to feel rather patronising. Consider the following anecdote:

---

* Taylor Arithmetic Frame is an assistive device for teaching arithmetic to visually impaired persons. The surface of its aluminium frame is divided into star-shaped holes with eight angles, thus allowing the double-ended metal types to be placed in different positions according to a set system.

'Your samosa is at three o'clock.' 'Oh no, your ice-cream is at nine.' I resisted his grip so that I could pinch my favourite jilebi at the bottom of my plate. 'That's at seven o'clock by the way.' Clearly, he was rehearsing a rehabilitation convention of naming objects* by their relative positions on a clock dial. I sensed him lean discretely towards my neighbour and whisper, 'You know, I need to be here until he is finished.' 'God is great.' 'They have people like us to take care.' I quickly wanted to get it done and over with. His unsolicited attention was making my favourite jilebi taste metallic and rusted. I must have swallowed it with all my might for sure.

What is the lesson this time around? Well, the art of description can also be a power game. The facility for description gives unrivalled power to those who have it. They can draw on the same for self-aggrandisement. 'You see, I am helping a blind man.' That kind of show-offishness. Is this perhaps the opposite of mothering? Consider this anecdote:

We were just back from a college tour. I had smuggled in a massive album. 'Do you want to describe the photos for me?' I remember asking. The idea was not to learn what the pictures were. I knew them by heart any way. I wanted that guy to know how high-spirited we were! 'A boy is standing.' 'Three girls are sitting.' Some more page flips 'Boys ... Girls ... Bench ... Lawn ...' 'Excuse me; I need to urgently meet my teacher.' I ran away escaping from what I now call crude literalism. God's punishment for showing off, I guess!

Make no mistake, crude literalism shapes much of our professional approaches to contemporary human conditions. There are doctors, for example, who may look at your x-ray report while writing up a quick prescription. Try asking them

---

* Standardised naming convention that minimises variation in descriptors.

about the content of the x-ray. You may hear at best some technical jargon. But this is not about doctor blaming. Most specialists, including specialists of the literary kind, consider expert knowledge as something that cannot be communicated without an esoteric vocabulary. I am sorry; they are mistaken. The stranger whom I cited above may well belong to this kind. Like many, he may have allowed himself to be seduced by the idea that some knowledge systems are untranslatable; especially for certain audiences. It is in this manner that photographs, medical diagnoses and avant-garde literary reflections remain tucked away for exclusive audiences.

My students and I have developed an antidote to this exclusivism. Let me call that approach 'Vala vala* pedagogy'. My students and I are simply great at this. Please ignore my hubris for a second. Sometimes I take a picture to class with me. 'What do you think about this picture?' Strange silence for a minute. 'Sir, there is an eagle flying around.' 'A kid can be seen on the ground.' Kinshuk kickstarted the discussion. 'What do *you* think, Karnalius?' 'Sir, it is a girl child; I can see a necklace.' 'She looks emaciated.' Suma and Priya chimed in. (These are my final-year students.) You may have already guessed what this discussion was all about. It had to do with Kevin Carter's famous photograph *The Vulture and the Little Girl.*†

---

* 'Vala vala' means aimless chatter in Tamil.

† *The Vulture and the Little Girl*, also known as *The Struggling Girl*, is a Pulitzer-prize winning photograph by Kevin Carter which first appeared in *The New York Times* on 26 March 1993. It is a photograph of a frail famine-stricken boy, initially believed to be a girl, who had collapsed in the foreground with a hooded vulture eyeing him from nearby. The child was reported to be attempting to reach a United Nations feeding centre about a half mile away in Ayod, Sudan (now South Sudan), in March 1993, and to have survived the incident.

A lot goes on when I ask my students to describe visual stuff to me. First, my students have this inner urge to offer a really esoteric, hi-fi description for their blind teacher. That's just the beginning though. They go on from there, bringing the picture alive three-dimensionally. Literal descriptions, opinions, political argumentation, sentimentalities, symbolic associations and the like follow. I would need many a page to record the lively discussions that follow. But there is a larger point I would like to make here. The art of description is an inherent trait. Given an opportunity, we would all like to speak. More importantly, we want our intervention to be of some use. All I need to do is to validate this inner urge. In return, my students end up doing a really fine job in describing pictures to me, their blind teacher.

To say that blindness is an optical condition is a truism. But there is much more to it than that. Blindness is also experiential knowledge. It can teach us so much about the art of description.

BOOK FOUR

Love's Labour

Note

Fierce love, moments of pure joy, a near spiritual effacing of the self and then the downside—that slow burn of grief, that deadly cocktail of anxiety, helplessness and anger, a sense of there being no end in sight, that smouldering, guilt-inducing resentment stemming from a life wrapped up in caring for a child with a disability, the things forgone, whether measures of progress, professional identities, financial stability, a sense of being part of a larger community, leisure or other relationships, the invisibility of care work and how gendered it often is ... How does one total it all? There is an absence of meaningful conversation around this area of human experience, a conversation that merits a whole other book really.

I have charted this overlooked terrain via conversations and personal accounts, one of which is mine. I knew Swati, Pramath, Sankaravadivelu, Shoba and Nimi from before and had had glimpses, fleeting or not so fleeting, of their struggles, their island-moments of happiness. But I had never had dedicated conversations with them on how their lives had been shaped by the presence of their children. Waheeda, Joyce and Mamtha were people I got to know in the course of writing this book.

We dwelled on what their lives had been like before the birth of their children up until the moment of 'diagnosis'. We spoke about the strategies they had discovered, the 'solutions' they had happened upon, the regrets they carry. They described to me their happiest moments and their most challenging ones. On their part, the conversations involved a difficult processing of experience, often a remembering of buried griefs. I am deeply grateful to them for the gift of their time, especially given how time-starved their lives are, and for the reflective nature of our conversations.

Swati and Pramath had to take turns talking to me so one of them could take care of their son, Karun. They spent over an hour each with me responding to my questions thoughtfully and meticulously, and always with a sense of responsibility. I met Waheeda at her small flat in Chennai. Her daughter Shameena was at home too that day, and was struggling with menstrual cramps. Waheeda did not wait for me to initiate the conversation, plunging instead into a narrative that flows easily and comes naturally to her. After all, it is the story of her life, a story she knows how to tell. Mamtha was not expecting me that afternoon but I allowed myself to be persuaded by her daughter, Chetna (also featured in this book), to visit her and her son, Tarak, at home. The conversation that happened was an impromptu one and was possible only because Chetna stepped in to take care of Tarak so that Mamtha could speak to me.

These conversations didn't happen together—at the same time and place—but given how connected they are, I have collaged them together so that they now appear as one big conversation.

They are followed by a personal account, also on the same theme.

Children Have to Be Delighted In

Conversations with Parents

Swati and Pramath are the parents of twenty-four-year-old Karun, who is on the autism spectrum. Swati worked for six to seven years at a research institute in India and is currently a full-time mother to Karun. Pramath teaches mathematics at an institute in Chennai.

Sixty-two-year-old Waheeda acts as primary caregiver to her daughter, Shameena, who is a thirty-five-year-old woman with an intellectual disability. Shameena spends three days every week at SAI Bakery, a neighbourhood initiative in south Chennai for adults with disabilities run by Sumithra Prasad (also interviewed for this book). Waheeda, who suffers from various health concerns herself, is finding it increasingly difficult to take care of her daughter. She is separated from her husband and lives with one of her sons.

Sankaravadivelu is the father of Diya, a young woman with a hearing impairment. He has an MA in English and a postgraduate diploma in management. He retired from service some years ago.

Shoba, Diya's mother, teaches in the kindergarten section of a Chennai-based school.

Ninety-one-year-old Joyce is the mother of fifty-year-old Babu who has Down's syndrome.

Mamtha is the mother of Tarak, a twenty-year-old with DAMP syndrome (Deficits in Attention, Motor control and Perception). She has volunteered at Vidya Sagar and provides informal support to parents of children with disabilities.

Nimi (name changed to protect identity) is a freelance translator. Her stepson Aditya (name changed to protect identity) was diagnosed with autism even before she married his father. Nimi was Aditya's primary caregiver until her divorce from his father some years ago.

What was your life like before your child was born? When did you first notice that something was amiss?[*]

Swati: I finished my PhD in the States and then returned to India. Pramath, my husband, was already back here. I was a postdoctoral fellow at an institute in Chennai. Eventually, we moved to Allahabad for professional reasons. That is where Karun was born. He was slightly behind in walking and more than slightly behind in talking for sure, but we figured it was because he was exposed to three languages at one go—Hindi, English and Telugu. Also, Pramath's mother spoke at age three. And so, we were not overly alarmed. Otherwise, he seemed fine. He seemed interested in the world around him. He would say certain words—car, for instance, or bus ... There was a small preschool for the children of employees on the institute campus and we started sending Karun there. One day, as I was walking home, a colleague from the institute, whose kids were slightly older than Karun (they were also in the same preschool), came running after me and said, 'Swati! Swati! You know what? Karun just doesn't listen!' As we talked about it, we agreed that this was also quite normal for that age. It bothered me, though, that this had alarmed her enough to draw my attention to it with that kind of urgency. Occasionally, the school would allow parents

---

[*] This question is not applicable to Nimi, given that she became part of her stepson Aditya's life only after he was diagnosed with autism.

to volunteer and spend time with the kids. That is when she had noticed that while she could get all the other children to participate in various activities, Karun would not. At some level, Karun's behaviour was age appropriate. Autism wasn't part of my vocabulary at the time. Karun would stack drums and play other games that did not require a partner. All toys, for Karun, were mechanical objects—not meaningful in an interactive world. One day, I was standing and watching out the window and this boy who was barely four or five months older than Karun was holding a bat while another kid was throwing a ball to him. The little boy was then hitting it back. Back then, I knew nothing about developmental stuff. But I knew in my heart that this activity was impossible for Karun.

Now I can say that it was not about hand-eye coordination or not understanding what the game was. What he didn't understand was why he should play such a game at all. First of all, to play such a game, you have to understand what the game is. And there is turn-taking involved. As opposed to rolling a car back and forth, where both people involved are doing the same thing, in this case, you are doing something different and I am doing something different. The action is far more complex in the sense that somebody is throwing a ball at you and you have to hit it with something. It seemed cognitively impossible for Karun, given that with him we could never even manage to get a game of throw and catch or roll something back and forth going. He had the coordination for it all. That was not the problem. But he just didn't see the *point* of it, because he didn't have the joint attention for it. We are doing this together; isn't that fun?—but he didn't get that. Games like these are about that occasional eye contact we make, that communicative instant we have. You don't play a game like this without making this connection, however momentary, with the other person. And he was capable of doing that, but just didn't see any point in it. However, I did not correlate this incident with the observation my colleague had made earlier. Nor did I think it was significant. I didn't think it would have such consequences or that it would be a lifelong issue. I merely assumed that Karun was a little behind, that he would catch up. Yet, a part of me—which I suppressed—wondered if this would ever happen. By and large, his interactions with us and other adults appeared normal. Looking back, his interactions with other children were negligible. Karun was two at the time. Sometimes other parents would come visiting, bringing with them their children. Karun knew these children. But he would drift away to the other room. And we would say, 'No, look, all the fun is *here!*'

When this happened recurrently, I thought it kind of odd. But I had never heard of autism. I didn't know. I hadn't a clue. I knew what it was to be mentally delayed. I could comprehend that, but it seemed that this was simply not the case with Karun because puzzles and so on he was able to do. There was a lot of understanding of language and even some meaningful speech. And you know, the look in the eye, you can tell—there was total comprehension of emotions and things. Once, when Pramath shouted at him and I said, 'aw', he didn't want that from me! He wanted Pramath to apologise! We would also play games around the bed—peekaboo or catch or running around the bed, though he was not too interested in reversing the roles, but still there was a lot of giggling and running around the bed and eye contact happening. There were plenty of good things also, so we were not too alarmed. So, we were really unable to join the dots. And join the dots and come to what conclusion? It was clearly not mental delay!

Karun was two when he was playing in a rainwater ditch and Pramath said, 'No!' to which Karun responded at once, 'You stupid!' He must have picked it up from playschool. It was so appropriate! Sometimes I would say, '*Karun, thoo tho buddhu hai!* (Karun, you are so naive!)' Then, I don't know how, he got the meaning of the word and once when I washed his hands forcibly, he called me a 'buddhu'. It was quite appropriate, you know. There was a lot of appropriate use of language and comprehension. So, we were not alarmed that way.

And then, when Karun was two and a half, we went to the US for a year. He went to the university daycare there. They had excellent facilities—even observation rooms with a one-way glass. Parents didn't have to sign or anything; they could just walk in to those rooms and watch the kids. No questions asked.

Karun cried the first six weeks. One day, I positioned myself in the observation room. As it happened, by some coincidence, he stopped crying and it looked like all our problems were solved. Speech and communication, however, had not quite taken off. Karun had also been thrown into a different language environment and a different culture. The university had a speech and audiology department. Sometime in December, they told us, 'Look, your son is almost three and isn't speaking yet. We can have him screened.' We thought, why not. I was finding it difficult to fill time when Karun was at home. We had the most beautiful house—a house on four levels, with swings and slides and a backyard. The people who left it to us (it was a sabbatical house) told us to go ahead and use their kid's clothes and toys. They gave us total freedom to use what was in the house. It was like a dream place and I still found it so difficult to fill time. Karun would be sitting on a swing, I would be pushing him and, you know, life should have been more fun, but it wasn't! But then, again, I had no clue. I didn't get alarmed or anything. I just thought, I don't know, we are boring people! Finally, the university did this screening. We then went for the last vacation I guess we had—to San Francisco.

Pramath: Karun's early years were spent in Allahabad. He seemed normal enough at the time. He used to go to this school on the campus. A friend of ours wandered into the school one day just to help the kids out and she told us, 'Karun doesn't listen.' That statement of hers struck a bell. A little later, when Karun was two years old, Swati went to Israel and I took Karun and went to Ahmedabad to visit my mother and brother. He flowered there. He was surrounded by relatives. My mother got some other kids to play with him. There was a nice garden. There was another girl. And I would ask myself—'Will Karun ever be like that?' I suppressed that thought. My mother hadn't started speaking until she was three and Karun was at least verbal at the time. So, it seemed like some things at least were going fine, that these other little signs were to be ignored. Two months later, we went to the US and he had a very hard time adjusting. I am sure I would have forgotten all this if everything had turned out okay.

Waheeda: My family is from Trichy. That's where I studied, but only till my ninth grade. My parents got me married to someone from Nagoor, near Nagapatinnam. He was working in the Electricity Board as an assistant engineer and was posted at Arakkonnam at the time. One year into my marriage, I got pregnant with Shameena. I went to my mother's house in Karaikal for my pregnancy. My parents were separated by then and my father had remarried, which is why my mother had come away to Karaikal. It was she who looked after me during my pregnancy. Shameena was born in the General Hospital. The delivery was a normal one. But after she was born, they didn't show Shameena to me. I was only told that I had had a baby girl. Later, they told me that because of the accumulation of phlegm in her lungs, they were giving her oxygen. When I returned to the room, I noticed that the baby looked a bit different. She was thin and very dark. I began to have doubts as to whether she was really mine. But they didn't warn us that there was a problem.

Sankaravadivelu: We had always wanted to have a child, a girl child, for whatever inexplicable reasons. I felt a girl child would be more affectionate. Shoba too felt the same. We decided to go in for an adoption because we did not want to go through the entire fertility treatment rigmarole. My friends had adopted a girl child at the time. So, we applied as well and were in the queue.

Shoba: This was after eleven years of marriage. We didn't want to adopt a child who was related to us. We wanted to adopt a child who didn't have a home or anyone to call her own, a girl child. Our friends had adopted a child from the Missionaries of Charity. We visited the place and liked what we saw and the way they did things. The rule back then was that you could formally adopt a child only after she had spent ninety days at home with you. So, we went back after this waiting period and decided to adopt her.

I was working at the time. The state government sent people to run a background check on us. We had first decided to adopt a child in June of 1997. In anticipation, I had quit my job. It was 1998 before we were actually able to complete the adoption process. I was thirty-eight years old at the time; Sankar (Sankaravadivelu) was not yet forty. Diya was born on 17 January 1998. She was a very tiny baby. She was a premature baby. Her birth weight was just a kilo and hundred grams. At three months of age, she weighed only two kilos and three hundred grams. She was very tiny. I used to have a dozen small feeding bottles because I had to give her frequent but small feeds. She could eat only small quantities of food at a time. After about forty minutes, she would throw up. And she did okay, generally. But in the nights, she would not sleep too well. She would wake up crying, struggling with chest congestion. Slowly, she got over all these issues.

Sankaravadivelu: As a small child, she was very active.

Shoba: Very naughty too!

Sankaravadivelu: Not naughty, just very active. We would put her in the crib or playpen because she would seek our attention all the time. She would jump up and down to catch our attention.

Shoba: That was mainly because of her impairment—she couldn't hear.

Sankaravadivelu: That's what we believe now.

Shoba: Yes, looking back that's what we think. She would cry but she never called out. In May 1999, Sankar was transferred to Cochin and we moved there.

Sankaravadivelu: We didn't realise this about Diya. We just assumed she would take some more time to talk.

Shoba: All her milestones were delayed—walking, sitting …

Sankaravadivelu: Her birth weight was low too. The thing is, the doctor didn't ask us to do the BERA test. She felt very bad about this later. She told us they usually do not approve

the adoption request without a BERA test but that this time
she had gone ahead and issued the approval. She had only
pointed out the low birth weight. We didn't realise there was
an issue at all. We kept expecting Diya to start speaking. But
then what she ended up with was fits.

Shoba: Because of her low birth weight.

Sankaravadivelu: We were really frightened. Shoba called
me. I rushed at once. We took Diya and ran to the hospital
behind our house. We found a very good paediatrician.

Shoba: She was from CMC Vellore. She instructed us to
give Diya an injection through the anus. We had to do this
whenever she got fits. The medicine would then go straight
into the nervous system. Diya got fits even with a mild fever.
This was all because of her low birth weight. The doctor also
advised us to sponge Diya down with cold water or place her
in a bucket of cold water whenever her temperature shot up,
but she would not allow us to do that. Around Diwali time,
my in-laws came down to Cochin for a visit. Just before
they visited—this was in September—we had gone over to
our friends' house, the same friends who had adopted a child
before us—Mahesh and Hema. We all went over to Mahesh's
in-laws' house. Diya was sitting on a swing and Mahesh's
mother-in-law called out to her. She kept on calling, 'Diya!
Diya!' but Diya did not respond. The lady didn't say anything
to us at that time. We returned home after lunch. It was only
later that Mahesh's mother-in-law told him, 'I may be wrong
but I repeatedly called Diya by name and she did not respond.'

Sankaravadivelu: I was in the office at the time. Mahesh's
mother-in-law called me directly. She knew something was
wrong.

Shoba: Diya was one year and eight months old at the time.

Sankaravadivelu: She said, 'Look, don't take this to heart,' and then told me what she suspected. She asked me to have it checked at once.

Joyce: We knew about Babu's condition—Down's syndrome—from when he was three months old. He wouldn't talk. He wouldn't do anything, wouldn't ask for anything. We had to somehow intuit his needs and act accordingly.

Mamtha: I grew up in Tambaram.* When I was still in school, I used to help my father with his medical shop. We lived on the first floor of a building. The ground floor was where our pharmacy was. Mine was a small world. Going to school, coming back home, helping my mother, helping my father out with the store—that used to be my routine. So, moving away from that familiar routine and shifting to Chennai was a huge change for me. But somehow, I got by, addressing the auto-drivers as 'anna' and trusting God. I appeared very bold and confident, but inside I had no idea of where I was going. I used to remember all the landmarks. My daughter was three and a half years old and my son was eleven months old. He would be constantly crying. Somehow, I managed. My husband is a businessman, and because of that he could not extend the level of support that was expected of him. For some reason, we didn't quite gel as well. He was around five or six years elder to me, and we got married, that's all. There was neither any understanding nor communication between us. I was only twenty-three when Tarak was born. I suspected that he was different somehow. He would keep crying. An irritability and incessant crying were constants. I reported this to the doctors and the fact that he would never imitate us or play with any toys. But the doctors were not ready to accept it.

---

* A suburb in Chennai.

When Tarak was about ten months old, the festival of Diwali came around. Loud crackers were being burst on the streets. We were just stepping out of an auto when I realised that Tarak was unconscious. His lips had started to turn a light purple. I called out to him and got no response. Only after some time did he gain consciousness. He started vomiting as well. I told myself that something was definitely wrong with the child. I took him to the doctor. All he said was, 'God has given you such a golden gift, a beautiful and chubby boy. Why are you constantly worrying about something?' There was this one time when I felt his breath stop. I then took him to another doctor. None of the doctors told me anything. Mothers should be informed correctly. That's the only way they can accept things and prepare for the future. Nobody told me this is going to be a lifelong challenge. Nobody gave me a heads up. When Tarak was about a year old, I consulted a neurologist close to my place. He didn't tell me anything either—just prescribed a CT scan, then referred me to an audiology clinic for a check-up. I took the CT scan, went to the audiology clinic. At the time, I couldn't read English too well, and neither could I comprehend the medical report. I used to have a lot of anxiety regarding these reports. It was the audiologist at the audiology clinic who suggested that I take Tarak to Spastic Society, to Vidya Sagar.

Tell me about the time you first received a proper diagnosis. How did you respond to it?[*]

Swati: We returned from our brief vacation to San Francisco to receive a report which said that even though Karun was

---

[*] This question is not applicable to Nimi, given that she became part of her stepson Aditya's life only after he was diagnosed with autism.

almost three, language-wise he was functioning at twelve–thirteen months. At first, we tried to dismiss it as jargon. We told ourselves that the expert who did the screening for Karun was required to submit a report and hence she had written one. But it troubled us enough that we requested to meet her. She explained that the issue was not a question of language or cultural difference. Karun wasn't able to understand the gesture—here she held up her palm in front of her—indicating 'give me this'. This is such a universal gesture, she told us, and I did not get a response from Karun. Her first child had Asperger's. He was fifteen then. That's why, I think, she had put so much effort into the report. Then she said, 'I am going to go out on a limb to say this—I am not qualified really to say the A word or give any diagnosis—but you should see a doctor. You need to have this checked.'

After we figured out what the issue was, we were overcome by a sense of deep despair. Karun too lost interest in life. It was like, I am not interested in life either if you are not interested in it. That was perhaps the reason why he did not respond to things like the snow. And even now, this holds. Karun's dependence on our moods is very high; he is so intuitive. He can guess my mood. This is one of the areas where emotional maturity has come to him. He can guess from the tone in which Pramath and I are talking to each other what we are feeling. The moment things start going off, he can pick up on it.

By the time we got the doctor's appointment, which was a good two months later, we had read enough that we had no doubt. Karun was half-asleep when we went to meet the doctor. She talked to us for a few minutes and then said, 'You *know*.' And we said, 'Yes, we do.'

Pramath: When we first received the diagnosis, it was devastating. We had no idea what to do. So many thoughts, all at the same time. One was sheer grief. There was also worry over the practical aspects. What was one supposed to do? What was next? I remember saying to the specialist as soon as she had pronounced her diagnosis, 'So that's that,' to which she responded emphatically, 'No, that's not that.' She said that there were many things we could do, starting then. But then we still had to pick Karun up from daycare. I think we picked him up early that day just because we felt protective towards him. I felt protective towards Swati too. The people we were working with, who we were supposed to spend a year with—our collaborators—we told them about Karun. They were very supportive. They spoke to the chair of the department. They found a way to keep us there one more year. Even though the official diagnosis took until May, one professor who had an autistic son was very helpful. We got our act together quickly, put Karun into speech therapy and so on.

Waheeda: Within forty days of her birth, my baby daughter developed hernia, then jaundice—all kinds of issues. We took her for treatment to the hospital and she was cured of all that. But they told us she was too weak at that point to be treated for hernia. It was then that they informed us that her brain was somewhat underdeveloped. They measured her head circumference and told us that her movements would be slow, that her IQ level would be stuck at age four, that she would be slow to develop. They advised us to take care of her and not be harsh. Be gentle with her, they said. She will do well then.

Sankaravadivelu: We took Diya to an ENT but he couldn't help us with a diagnosis. He suggested that we go to

Trivandrum, where we could get a BERA test done. We took her there, but they were not able to do much there either. Then we went to Bangalore and met her paediatrician. She suggested a place but there too we didn't get much help. Then she asked us to go to Mysore, to the All India Institute for Speech and Hearing.

The testing process was difficult.

Shoba: Yes, Diya was not supposed to move during the test. They sedate the children.

Sankaravadivelu: Yes, they make sure they are not awake and only then do they perform the procedure. We stayed in Mysore for a day. They had to repeat the test twice. Then they concluded ...

Shoba: Profound hearing loss ...

Sankaravadivelu: Profound hearing loss ... that was the diagnosis. Our paediatrician was literally in tears. She put us on to another developmental paediatrician. This lady was very good. She said we didn't have to worry. She told us, 'You have only one choice but it is a very good choice. Take her to Bala Vidyalaya in Chennai.' Diya was not yet two. We did all of this in under a month. In December I sent Shoba and Diya straight from Bangalore to Chennai. I was still in Cochin. I called my cousin and told him what the problem was. This cousin helped us a lot. We admitted Diya to Bala Vidyalaya immediately.

Shoba: It was just before the Christmas break. I was told by the teachers at Bala Vidyalaya that the school would reopen on 18 January. This was in the year 2000. Diya's birthday falls on 17 January.

Joyce: When Babu was around ten years old, we took him to a hospital outside the city. The doctor who checked him told us that his brain growth was very limited and that he would always behave like a small child. He wouldn't behave like a grown up and his brain would not grow beyond the capacity of a ten-year old's. They asked us to enrol him at a special school.

Mamtha: I took Tarak to Vidya Sagar when he was eleven months old. I started very early. It was all God's grace. I remember it all vividly. When the doctor was done with his assessment, I was holding one child in one hand and the other child in the other.

What things did you try in the early years?* What 'solutions' did you come up with?

Swati: The first thing we did was to put Karun into speech therapy. He really responded to what we did with him that year. A year later we started him on something called ABA— Applied Behavioural Analysis therapy. This therapy was initiated by a mother who had put her own daughter through it and 'rescued' her from autism. It was like dog training. If they got eight out of ten questions or activities right, that was seen as success and it was rewarded. If not, they were punished. There was a lot of repetitiveness to it. Tell me, which normal child will sit there and take the monotony of that? It may have been fine to get the initial foot in the door when the kid is not learning anything. It may work for a limited time—half an hour or an hour in a day. But it was touted as the only scientifically proven method that worked. Don't even ask me now what the data showed. I don't want to revisit that. So basically, the child would just sit there and had to

---

* This question is not applicable to Nimi, given that she became part of her stepson Aditya's life only after he was diagnosed with autism.

soak in it all day. I put my foot down in two hours. But I think that therapy really set Karun back. Then we moved to Canada, where it was much easier to access ABA than speech therapy. It was free for children who qualified to receive this therapy. ABA was the road most parents took. It is important to do natural, simple things with your children. You don't have to torture them! ABA, for Karun, was torture. My gut was screaming out against it. But I said, okay, what to do, this is what I am told. In fact, a mother who had tried this therapy with her son (and claimed he had actually recovered) equated it with surgery that is necessary and good for the child. When you draw that analogy, what else can you do?

Waheeda: For a long time, we didn't know what to do. It was a while before we acted. My husband wasn't supportive. He was embarrassed by Waheeda's presence and never spoke to her kindly. At some point, his elder brother suggested a school in Chennai. He admitted Shameena to a hostel there. After a month, they sent her home for vacation. Unfortunately, the principal of the school passed away and it had to be shut down. The school was really good. They would take the kids out. It was Shameena's ill luck, really.

None of the other schools worked out. Shameena is slow even when it comes to eating. The others at SAI bakery have progressed so much—Babu and Richard talk a lot. The others do too. Only Shameena remains sitting there silently. I must tell them that sometime. Sahitya used to talk to her a lot. But he fell sick. So, they don't want to put any strain on him.

Shoba: Bala Vidyalaya told me that before the school reopened, I should make sure Diya was fitted with a hearing aid. 'Don't bring her without that,' they said. They gave me an address. We fitted her with the hearing aid. For the first time she began hearing sounds! She would get irritated, pluck the hearing aid from her ears and throw it away. She didn't know what it all meant!

Sankaravadivelu: Small child—she didn't know …

Shoba: 18 January, the first day of school. Diya had just turned two. She was hearing sound for the first time and she didn't like it. She didn't know what the sounds were, what they meant. She could not even recognise her own crying. So, it took a long time … During the Christmas vacation, it took me a long time to get her used to the hearing aids. The school told us to talk to her only in English since we were planning to get her educated in the English medium. We were not to substitute an English word with words from any other language. We were not allowed to even use the Tamil word 'kadugu' for mustard. So, it was a real process of learning for me. We say so many things in our vernacular language but I had to use English for everything.

Shoba: At school, they told us not to use any gestures while talking to the child. Normally, everyone uses gestures. But in Diya's case, we could only use speech. There was no question of sign language. Also, we were not, under any circumstance, to visit another hearing-impaired child's home because then the children would start signing to each other. They would make up their own signs while the parents were talking. I followed that instruction to the T.

Sankaravadivelu: We were not supposed to watch television either.

Shoba: Yes, because the children would not listen to the audio, they would only look at the visuals. They were not trained for audio … At Bala Vidyalaya, we started with one hour of classes.

Sankaravadivelu: Shoba had to go along with Diya and stay through the day.

Shoba: Diya was at Bala Vidyalaya for four years and six months. For the first three years, I used to accompany her and stay by her side. I have her report card. I can show it to you. She did not take leave even for a single day. She had full attendance!

Sankaravadivelu: It was a very tough job. Every day, Shoba had to go along to school, teach Diya everything ...

Shoba: We had to go on talking to her ... None of these children had heard sound before. They had no vocabulary. So, when you went out with them, you had to say, 'Look, this is a tree. What is a tree? Its trunk is brown, the leaves are green.' You had to talk, talk, talk ...

Sankaravadivelu: Especially the sounds of birds, animals. We had to mimic the sounds they made. Sometimes we had to buy bird and animal toys to teach her.

Shoba: We had to take her out to many places—to the children's park, to the fire station, to the zoo ... I think she has seen those sea lions four times! It is all about exposure. That's what helps the children.

Joyce: We enrolled him in a school in Madurai. He studied there for seven years, after which they said they couldn't keep him anymore. It was a co-ed school, a regular school. It was called Anbagam then, but I don't know what it is now. He studied there until he was seventeen. We kept him at home after that and I tried teaching him. He could not speak, couldn't say words. He at least speaks one or two words now.

Mamtha: For me, taking him to Vidya Sagar is what felt right. If I hadn't done that, I would have lost my son. At least he's mobile now. Everything was delayed—there was global delay and milestone delay. It is only because I took a few decisions against my family's wishes that he is mobile right now. He's able to communicate. He used to move on his butt, which resulted in rashes. He did not have any concentration. Vidya Sagar was a place where I learnt so many things. I remember hardly having any relationship with others in the family at that time, not even with my husband. I would just about cook, that's all. Every evening would be used up in occupational therapy. Whatever they did at school, we would have to do all over again for another hour. I didn't know much about it; I just followed what I was told to do blindly. But I felt the early intervention programme was helping. I saw so much progress.

Baking as a part of occupational therapy, speech therapy— all of this was very new to me. My first teacher was Kavitha. She was a young physiotherapist with a lot of patience. I did not have that kind of patience. She would scold me and say, 'Sometimes be a mother too! Why are you always like a teacher?' Every toy or doll I came across would set me thinking as to how I could make it a teaching aid. I wanted to teach Tarak everything, so he could do his best. I even neglected my daughter in the process. I would always tell her, 'You have to play with bhaiya.' She didn't realise all this when she was small. Only when she reached eighth or ninth grade did she realise something was wrong. Even I did not realise I was robbing her of her childhood. I was insisting that she play with her brother. I did not realise that she was not living her childhood, and that it would never return. I think that was a mistake on my part. She was very responsible. She would go to her tuitions all by herself; she would ask the traffic police to help her if she had to cross the road. I placed a whole lot of responsibilities in her hands. In the process, she grew really mature. Other parents would often ask me how I dared to send my daughter out on her own. They would always drop and pick up their children. I feel that approach has helped her in taking strong decisions. I kept all teaching materials at home. I decided to refrain from spending on luxuries. Somewhere between the ages of seven and nine, Tarak started sight reading. He could clearly identify around twenty-five to thirty words. I was really enthused observing his progress, but I felt that it took him a really long time to learn academic stuff. I never compared him with other children. In any case, each of these children had a different sort of disability.

I always get my son to help me with things. I tell him to fetch water, for instance, or to put the dishes in the sink. And I praise him for his help so that he feels happy, so that he knows he is actually helping. I have also learnt—as a parent—that the child will keep changing. I tell other parents not to be too fixated. For instance, just because the child is doing some sight reading now, one should not put him into regular school immediately. If you do that, then everything is lost and you begin to feel depressed again. It is important that the child learns basic life skills and self-care before anything else.

Some things are difficult to teach, like the whole issue of sexuality, for instance. I started to place a few pillows between Tarak and me and told him, 'This is your place, this is my place. You should sleep there.' Even then, he would try to put his legs over me or touch me. When he turned fourteen, I told him that he must sleep away from me. If you ask him to hug or kiss someone, he will do it. It is nothing for him. But not every person would like that, right?

What has been the hardest part of all this? What happened to other aspects of your life, professionally, for instance? How did being the parent of a child with a disability change things? What sort of roadblocks did you face— with school/college, with the treatments or the therapies that you tried?

Swati: Pramath was away on a ten-day work trip to Germany when I was officially informed by the supervisor that the data showed that Karun was not responding positively to the therapy. He more or less agreed with my assessment that Karun was nothing like the child who was first taken to them. I began to fall apart and had my first panic attack in the few days that I was alone with this bad news. The day after my meeting with the supervisor, I dropped Karun off at preschool, came home, made a cup of a tea and found myself bawling. I couldn't stop. In an hour's time, I had to drive a short distance to get him from school. While driving there, I had my first panic attack. I had to pull over and park for a while because my body had gone all limp. When I got to school, I told the teacher I couldn't trust myself at the wheel. The teacher then dropped Karun and me home. Pramath could not be reached over the phone. I called up the airlines and got them to change Pramath's tickets. Karun and I spent the intervening days in the house of a distant relation. Pramath returned earlier than planned. I have had panic attacks off and on since then.

We spent a fortune on ABA over a period of ten months. We were slow in applying for state funds and, in any case, there was a waitlist. During this time, we watched Karun steadily go into a decline in every way. He became a withdrawn, depressed child, whereas earlier he had blossomed in response to the therapy he had been receiving. The supervisor of the behavioural therapy kept trying to get us to stick with the programme but I didn't want to. We then enrolled Karun in a speech-based therapy but it was difficult to find a speech therapist who would come home. By then, Karun had been badly hurt by ABA and was a different child. He wasn't going to respond to speech therapy the way he had the first time around. There was a centre that offered behavioural therapy in a more natural, school-like setting. This centre was headed by a speech therapist and we felt that it was the only option available at the time. We could not get a home-based therapist and we needed a team. We paid the centre a lot of money but at least there was some social interaction. Financially, we were drained by this process. After about two years of this, we felt Karun was not getting anywhere. I went to a number of occupational therapists but that only made a marginal difference. Something was wrong with our approach.

Pramath: Karun's presence in my life has changed it enormously. I can't even imagine what life would have been had Karun been normal. I have a certain distance from it all may be, compared to Swati. But it is only relative—only because I get to get away. I can chat about mathematics and this and that, whereas Swati doesn't get that space. I wouldn't say I have recovered. There is always a general anxiety, a desire to protect Karun. To make sure that we give him not just what he needs for comfort but that he gets to enjoy some things, that he cracks a certain code in this mysterious world. Why, I don't know. But I feel a sentient being should have that. It is my responsibility to ensure that. Maybe it is a deeper attachment. Sometimes I say that he is like a muggle caught in a world of wizards. I don't think I ever mentally relax and that has taken its toll. Swati relaxes even less than I do. I gave up research, in a sense, for there were many things to do. Then we moved to Canada and I was looking for a job, so I resumed research. Except, I started doing longer research projects. Pragmatic considerations should have meant shorter and more papers, but I can't force things anymore because so much of my energy goes elsewhere; so when it comes to research I just have to go with what the inner call is.

Waheeda: Shameena gets lazy. I sometimes ask her to do some household chore or the other. Then she will do it. But she won't do it on her own. Even television is something she won't watch on her own. If she gets some exercise during the day, she sleeps well at night. But otherwise, she doesn't sleep and is then restless during the day. I am not able to cope these days. I would like to admit her to a home if possible. Once, my son suggested that I take a break and go with him to Bangalore for two days. My daughter-in-law was left in charge of Shameena. But Shameena can be quite stubborn. When I was away, my daughter-in-law requested Shameena to close the balcony door because she didn't want her one-and-a-half-year-old son, my grandson, to fall from the balcony when she was not watching. But Shameena refused and continued sitting in the balcony. As it happened, my daughter-in-law went to use the restroom. In the meantime, my grandson crawled up to the balcony and stuck his head in the railing. My daughter-in-law had a tough time extricating him. I rushed back from Bangalore. So that's how it is.

Shoba: Academically, Diya has always been above average. Again, college admission was quite a challenge. Students at Ananya Learning Centre typically sit for the NIOS exams. These results are usually declared very late.

Sankaravadivelu: I had to run to the university, get Diya exempted from second language. They were quite helpful there. I had to go to the Madras Medical College to get a certificate declaring that Diya was hearing-impaired so that the university would give us the exemption. We had to run the BERA test on her. They made a small error in spelling her name on the certificate, but we managed that issue somehow. We also managed to get her into a college in Chennai.

Shoba: It was not very easy. They are not aware that these children can do well.

Sankaravadivelu: Firstly, these children need smaller class sizes. Secondly, you need some specialised teachers to handle them and to train other teachers as well. There are children with various other impairments. The involvement of parents is very important too.

Shoba: We don't have learning support in India for different kinds of learners.

Sankaravadivelu: For instance, these children should be trained only in basic math.

Shoba: When Diya was in her first year of college, her tourism and travel course required that you had to learn a foreign language—German. We explained to them that it was a one-language system as far as Diya was concerned. They said that was okay, that she could just sit in on the classes, since there were credits for that course. I told them she wouldn't be able to manage. We paid up for the course but she could not manage! She could not pass the exam. She felt so bad. The foreign language for the second year was Japanese. I told them she would not enrol for it, that she didn't need the credits.

Sankaravadivelu: The certificate had clearly exempted her. When I pointed that out to them, they finally exempted her from foreign language. They didn't have an alternative course to offer her though. This was only meant to be an extra course—to enhance their skills ...

Sankaravadivelu: Later, they discovered she was good with word processing, she could type. They gave her work like that during language class.

Shoba: She used to enjoy that. The class strength in college was seventy. That was a huge disadvantage ...

Sankaravadivelu: Given the fact that Diya has a certificate stating that she is hearing-impaired from the National Institute of Speech and Hearing, they should have helped her out. She cannot learn the way normal children can. Such children need help even when it comes to jobs. There are, of course, some very bright children who have hearing impairments. There is one child like that who has made it to IIT!

Shoba: The mother of that child identified the issue when her daughter was very young. She had dropped a heavy vessel within earshot of the child, who hadn't jerked at all. That was when she found out. The child was only twenty-eight days old at the time.

Sankaravedivelu: One parent had to dedicate himself or herself fully to looking after Diya. I was in Cochin, paying a high rent. After some time, I felt it was going to be difficult. The priority was to get Diya to speak. I quit my job and came away to Chennai. We then moved here to Thiruvanmiyur. Initially, Shoba and Diya stayed with my cousin in Kilpauk. Shoba would commute by auto all the way to Bala Vidyalaya. She would hold Diya all the way, Diya would fall asleep. Poor thing, she was a small child ...

Shoba stayed there for six months. Then I said enough is enough. It was a very difficult time for us. My career had gone for a toss and we didn't know what was going to happen to Diya, what the road ahead was. Of course, we also had to save money. We had some money so we were able to support ourselves. Then I took up a job with a much lower salary.

Shoba: The school was completely free. That was its beauty.

Sankaravadivelu: But we had savings, so there was no problem. We didn't really have to ask anyone for help. But we had to scale down our lifestyle. Before this problem surfaced, we used to eat out very often. We gave up all that. Diya was very small; she didn't feel the lack of all this. She was a happy, active child. In Cochin, we had an apartment on the twelfth floor. We used to keep all the doors shut. Diya usually stayed in the playpen. We had a cook and a maid. We lived a very good life. One day, we found that Diya was missing! Shoba searched everywhere and finally we found that she had climbed out of the playpen and was hanging from the balcony window. We rushed and held her.

Joyce: It was only after twenty-eight years that Babu spoke a little. He never used to even say 'Amma' or 'Appa'. He continued to stay at home and wouldn't do as he was told. He would run away often. When he was seventeen years old, he disappeared. Somebody took him away. The people who harvest organs—eyes, kidneys, etc.,—they took him away. We were devastated for the next three days. We cried a lot. We were extremely worried about him. We advertised on TV and papers. We even put up posters everywhere. We got information on the third day saying he was at a certain place. Immediately, the children in our house, including my sister-in-law's sons, went and brought him back safely. After that we kept him only at home. We were very scared to send him anywhere after that.

Mamtha: Sometimes, people ask me what I have to show for all these years with regard to Tarak. Then, I feel like crying. We have given our lives for this. I have observed every movement of my son's, every single nerve. I used to think deeply about each of his behaviours. I didn't play the other roles I was supposed to play—that of a mother to my daughter, that of a wife, that of a daughter. I have only been a mother to Tarak.

Nimi: Finding a playschool for Aditya was hard. In Calicut, there were schools willing to take him but they didn't know what to do with him. There were some special schools too but my former husband's family wasn't very happy about sending him there. I finally found a school that I thought would be good for Aditya because it had a large ground and the teachers were friendly. But it was not a posh school. When Aditya's father came and saw the school, he wasn't very happy. Nor was my mother-in-law. She said, 'I heard you found some low-class school for Aditya.' That was the most difficult thing about it all—how to please the family, how to make them understand. In this school, they kept saying Aditya is deaf. They didn't quite understand. The teacher kept saying we should take him to an ENT and correct his hearing. It was so difficult for me to explain to them, to get them to understand that it wasn't deafness that was the issue ...

I would say Aditya's absence of social skills was really difficult for me. If I took him to someone's house, he would just barge in, go into the kitchen, open the cupboard, open the fridge, help himself to chocolate ... We couldn't take him out to houses where we didn't know the people too well. Aditya used to grab mobile phones from people who came home. All that I found very difficult. I found it hard to control him.

Tell me about the interventions that you have tried, the ones which you find have worked.[*]

---

[*] There were no responses from Mamtha and Joyce to this question.

Swati: I found this remarkable therapist who taught us how to 'thaw' Karun out. She would come home. She charged ninety-five dollars per visit and would make these three-hour long visits. She would keep at it until she felt she had achieved something. It was wonderful to have someone who was not watching the clock. She would even follow him to the closet and sit on the floor if she had to, to work with him. She taught us a lot. Behavioural therapy doesn't work beyond a point. The child stops caring. Then you have to say, here's a human being, we have to meet him halfway. Why is it not working? The speech therapist taught us—here's a human being, you have to see that. They have real feelings, they get hurt. So, you have to watch for that. This lady worked with Karun for two years until we left Canada for the US. It was a big thing in my life. I learnt so much from watching her. She was over fifty at the time.

Waheeda: I have two daughters and three sons. My second son, Mubrarak, is in the US. A friend of his told him about SAI—Sumithra and Sai bakery. He told him that they would take good care of Shameena. After speaking to Sumithra, I felt confident that my daughter had a place in this world. Sumithra addressed Shameena when she spoke. That was really nice. She told me it was important that we respect Shameena, that we give her the feeling that we like her. Shameena got very attached to Srini, Sumithra's son. Srini was also very fond of her. He used to read to her. Shameena can't read but is very interested in books. Srini would make her sit next to him and keep talking to her. So, she started speaking as well. Sumithra told me about speech therapy too. Shameena started to bloom. She started to smile, to look happy. But at home, the moment she saw her father, it was a different story. She would grow all quiet. I used to accompany Shameena to SAI bakery. But her father wanted me at home so I could make him coffee. He instructed me to send her there by share-auto. But I couldn't send her alone since she doesn't speak. My husband married again at this time and I came away here to Adayar. So, for some time, Shameena couldn't go to SAI bakery. Then Lakshmi, a well-wisher and volunteer at SAI, arranged for an auto and a reliable driver. Now, I send Shameena thrice a week. There's been no problem since then.

Unlike the others though, she hasn't picked up any skills or activities. She will colour, arrange and sort the vegetables, pack cookies inside a box and so on. But unless you tell her to do something, she won't. She can't read or process text. If you point out specific pictures to her and explain what they represent, then she usually comprehends. She understands everything but cannot speak properly. She is thirty-six now but cannot express herself properly.

Shoba: Vidya Mandir, the school that Diya went to after Bala Vidyalaya, gives a lot of importance to children with disabilities such as Diya's. They are used to handling them. When she went for her interview, they were happy that she was able to read. She had never learnt the alphabets. They don't teach them that at Bala Vidyalaya. She learnt this only in grade one.

Sankaravadivelu: But she could read any book at all. Today, she doesn't read that much. She used to read really fast in those days.

Shoba: On her first day at Vidya Mandir, Diya wore a school uniform for the first time. I had asked her to observe the other children and do as they did. Diya was a very independent child. When I went to pick her up, I could see that she had cried. There were tear marks on her face. I asked her what happened. She said, 'You had told me to do as the others did. They were crying and so with great difficulty I too cried!' I didn't know whether to cry or to laugh! She made a lot of friends in Vidya Mandir. They would include her in everything. She even became a girl guide. She was doing quite well.

Nimi: When Aditya was about fourteen, I found him one day wearing one pair of shorts over another and looking very restless and uncomfortable. Initially, I didn't know what the issue was but later I understood that he was experiencing an erection and not being sure how to deal with it, was actually quite frightened. I was then told by his teachers that I should get his father to speak to him. But his father refused to do any such thing. He was quite sure Aditya wouldn't get any of it. I still remember sitting on the terrace and explaining to Aditya that his father too experienced what he was JUST beginning to experience and that it was alright, that he should go to his bedroom whenever he felt that way. This made such a difference to Aditya! His fear vanished. Just imagine how much easier it would have been had his father done the explaining!

How did the rest of the family respond to the situation?

Swati: At first, they couldn't believe it—just like everyone else. When Karun was about four, we visited my family. My grandmother noticed that he kept repeating things over and over. She said so. My parents did not respond to her remarks and I did not know how to tell her. My parents knew but they didn't know it was a lifelong condition. They thought he would outgrow it just like we had outgrown things in the past.

Pramath: My mother passed away a month before Karun was diagnosed. My brother was extremely concerned. He spent that summer with us. Swati's parents only got to know later. Her siblings were extremely supportive. I don't know what they went through in their heads, but both families were very supportive. Swati's brother was in Chicago. He too spent time with us. We had a lot of family visiting in those days, much more than we do now.

Waheeda: My husband didn't like the baby at all. One reason for this was that she was a girl. He had been transferred to Tirunelveli at the time. He was there for two years. He didn't come to visit us after that. When he came to the hospital to see her the first time, he was shocked. Because the baby was dark, he insisted that the nurse must have switched her at birth. He blamed my mother and lost his temper with me. After that, he didn't visit us at all. On the fortieth day, my in-laws had a small celebration, a function for the baby. They forced him to attend this but he was still not happy. He was worried, refused to talk to us, didn't hold the baby. He rejected her outright. As she grew older, he would say over and over again, 'This is not my child, Di. They must have switched her at birth.' But the thing is, she resembled her dad so closely. She had his face! My mother-in-law supported me all through this. She kept telling my husband, 'Look, she is your child.' But he wouldn't listen. I carried on as best as I could. My mother-in-law and sister-in-law were supportive and the baby did quite well. I was twenty-two when Shameena was born. My husband was planning to work in Saudi Arabia at the time. He even managed to go there but had to return because of some problems. He stayed home for a year with no work. He blamed his ill luck on the child. Two years later, in 1986, my first son was born. Then things began to look up for my husband. But he continued to reject Shameena. He wouldn't speak to her and would ask me to keep her locked up when we had visitors. He left for Saudi once again. Two or three years later, he sent for me. He was finding it difficult to cook. I took Shameena along with me. Shameena was barely eight when she attained puberty. Her father would torture her a lot—he would beat her up, shout at her. I tried very hard to manage the situation but couldn't bear to see her suffer. So, I left her with my mother in Trichy. My mother took care of her. She even tried to get Shameena enrolled in a school, but nothing worked. The children in special schools were in very bad shape. My mother was advised to train Shameena at home, which she did quite well. She even managed to get her to speak. But she didn't give her any work to do, as a result of which she grew lazy. Shameena was then sent to my mother-in-law's house and she stayed there for a while. Shameena has no other problem. She can speak, she can comprehend what others say. But she is scared of her father and this creates a problem. She understands perfectly when he says, 'Why do you want to keep her alive? Why don't you just kill her?' Even though Shameena is terrified of her father, she is also fond of him. Her fear of him has made her worse, which is why she doesn't speak at all.

Sankaravadivelu: It was a big shock to them. They were worried about how we would tackle it. But when we started doing things, when we started addressing the issue, they left us to it. We could never attend family functions. But no one questioned us.

Shoba: They were supportive of us. There was never any pressure to visit them.

Sankaravadivelu: We were not able to travel. We were completely tied down ...

Joyce: My husband used to keep Babu at home. He was protective of him, very affectionate towards Babu. My other children, including my brother and sister's children—everyone loves him. He is the last person of his generation. I have nine siblings. I was the tenth child in my family. So, he is the last child among all his cousins, and everyone likes him a lot. Babu this, Babu that ... they get him anything he asks for.

Mamtha: My husband is a very quiet person. He would wake up in the morning, eat, set off for his shop, return late in the evening, eat his dinner and then fall asleep. He is generally quite supportive. He is quite ready to eat idlis or bread and milk when I am unable to cook anything else. When I started taking Tarak to Vidya Sagar, he began to think that it would not be a lifelong condition. Then, one day, I told him, 'Look, your son is never going to be able to take care of your business, alright? This isn't that sort of a disability. It is a lifelong thing. We have to support him.' So, slowly, he started to accept it. I asked the people at Vidya Sagar to counsel and involve fathers as well. They arranged for a meeting with all the fathers and my husband too attended it. It was then that he began to understand. He had been watching me run around to so many places, manage so many things. He understood it all very well. I would burn the idlis at times. Many times, I would fall asleep in the evenings after working with Tarak. My husband would be standing outside, waiting to be let in. He would try knocking, even try throwing the bricks meant for Tarak's brick-walking on the door and call out. After that meeting at Vidya Sagar, he understood that Tarak's was a lifelong condition and he started to help out. If a customer came to his shop and asked, 'Brother, do you have diapers for big children?', he would ask them, 'How old is your child?

What is the problem?' And then he would tell them, 'I also have a son with special needs. Here, this is my wife's number. You can speak to her. She has been helping my son. I don't know much but she can be of help.' He would then hand me the customer's number. He would always remember to ask me later, 'Did you speak with them? So what if they haven't called? You can call and help them out.'

Nimi: I think nobody really understood what it was, actually. My parents didn't know much about it so they didn't say much either. But people who knew what autism was all about responded differently. One of my aunts said, 'Be very careful. It is a big responsibility, make sure somebody is there to take care of this child.' I was prepared for Aditya as I had taught in a special school before, seen children with autism. But I wasn't prepared for the reaction of my former husband's family.

You must have a sense of your child's inner life. What do you think goes on in his/her mind?*

Pramath: Karun has an inner life, yes. Can I articulate that? No, I can't. I certainly believe that Karun knows he is different. At least as he presents himself, his world revolves around his parents and music. He is still trying to crack the code; I think he speculates about the larger world, wonders about his place in the scheme of things. I suspect he asks himself how other people are so sure about their place in the world and how come he is not. Karun has very few pleasures. The whole point, from his point of view, is to still the many things in his head. Not just sensory things. It is an underlying anxiety about a difficult world. As he is growing older, maybe

---

* There were no responses from Joyce, Mamtha and Nimi to this question.

he wonders—projects himself into the future—I sense that. Surely, he used to wonder about the other kids like him. I have seen him hurt by something I said. You can say this happens with every child. But I think it is as sophisticated as older people being hurt. The question was: Do I know what his inner life is ... Karun takes satisfaction in music, relates to its mood. He is touched by it. There is an inner life. It is gratifying but also scary. It means he can also get depressed, and he does. There is a human being there, and I don't just mean that in the romantic sense. I am unable to articulate the larger picture he has in his mind. But to work with him, I have to make a mental model of him.

Waheeda: I can't make out what is going on in Shameena's mind. But if we lose our cool with her and speak to her in raised voices, she gets angry. When she is on her period, she tends to get even more angry. She is not able to tell us when she suffers from menstrual cramps. Her teacher has asked us to handle her with care. I even enquired about the possibility of a hysterectomy. One doctor I spoke to refused flatly. She struggles so much when she is on her period. She doesn't quite understand what is going on. But the doctors say that a hysterectomy could lead to side effects such as leg pain.

Shoba: Diya always says, 'I can hear. Only in the night I can't hear because you make me remove the hearing aids.' She never feels she has a problem. When we are travelling, she does not like to remove her hearing aids in front of others. She does not think of herself as someone with a problem.

Sankaravadivelu: Also, she doesn't consider herself as an adopted child. So, she has no problem about that either.

Shoba: Yes, she always says, I am thin like my father. I have horrible hair like my mother.

Sankaravadivelu: There are children who may think a lot about the fact that they are adopted. But Diya is not bothered at all. We don't have to worry about that.

Shoba: Only one day when she was young, she came home in the evening and asked me, 'So there's another amma and appa?' That was a shock for me. Maybe something had come up in school. She then asked me where her biological parents were. I said I didn't know. Then she asked, 'Why did they leave me?' I said, 'Maybe they were not able to take care of you.' After that, until today, she has not asked me about them.

Sankaravadivelu: We took her to Missionaries of Charity in Bangalore once. She saw the children there and started to cry. She said, 'Appa I want to go. I don't want to be here.'

Shoba: They advised us not to take her back there again. They were happy she had grown so attached to and identified with us.

Could you describe for me your happiest moments as a parent, your moments of joy—either because of some progress that the child has made or because of a shift in terms of how you started to perceive things and your role as a parent?*

Pramath: Plenty of moments of joy. Progress—yes, progress brings joy. But there is something instantaneous about moments of joy—it is just connections made with Karun. Extreme affection shown by him, for instance. Or when he takes pleasure in something in a way that suggests an inner life—to use your term—and you see that he has taken pleasure in that. To give you an example, there was a time in 2002 or 2003; it was winter and we were out walking

---

* There was no response from Mamtha to this question.

across a bridge. It was a nice day, cold and beautiful, in a place called Mississauga, a suburb of Toronto. We stopped for a while and the sun was setting. It was beautiful in the way that only winter days can be. Indescribable in a sense. Karun was transfixed by the beauty and he just stared. Then he looked at me to share that moment, and looked back at the sun. I don't think we can see that as progress, but a moment of joy—to think that both of us were looking at something—he was taking pleasure in it and was sharing it with me, a certain synergy in the joy. In early spring, we were in a town called Burlington. We walked up a hill from which there was a gorgeous view of Lake Ontario. Karun just ran up the hill, pointed at it—that exact point at the lake—and returned to us with a 'Did you see that?' kind of look. Both Swathi and I were thrilled about it. A third example ... Karun was extremely close to a babysitter in Indiana. She came to visit us in Mississauga. I don't think we told Karun she was coming. He was thrilled to see her. Then he did something interesting. He told me to go away from the room. 'Daddy, go do the blender,' he said. He kicked me out and closed the door. And then, after playing with her for some time, he felt he had to do something to compensate for shooing me away. Which is a very tough thing for an autistic child because they don't have a theory of mind.

Waheeda: When Shameena laughs and appears happy, I feel happy too. If they take her out to a sports meet and so on, she feels really happy. It is only at home that she starts looking dull. My son always spends some time with her. My daughter-in-law does too. But she does not give her too much time. Shameena fights a lot with my youngest daughter. 'I don't want Noora,' she will say. I tell her, 'But Noora likes you!' Shameena is fond of my son because he takes her out now and then. When she comes home, I always ask what she did that day at school. After a lot of nudging and prompting, she will say a few words.

Shoba: Diya is very independent. Never gives up. When a knot is tied tight, she will not rest until it is removed. That makes me happy.

Sankaravadivelu: She is also very stubborn. That's the other side. When I was away from Chennai for some years, my absence affected her a lot. So, I grew soft towards her.

Shoba: She knows how to get things done. If there's something she wants, she will just inform Sankaravadivelu that she already has my permission! She only informs us, never asks! She is very close to her grandparents. She helps them a lot.

Sankaravadivelu: She is very sensitive. Loves animals. Unfortunately, we can't take care of a dog here. The doctor advised us to adopt a pet but that will be difficult.

Joyce: Babu usually listens to everything I say, but sometimes he gets on my nerves. I beat him when he does something wrong but he will smile right through that! If I ask him, 'Why are you doing this, Babu? Why do you make Amma angry?', he will simply say, 'No, no.' He can't get the words right. He also loves going to church. There is nobody in church who doesn't enquire after Babu. When he doesn't come, everyone asks why he isn't there. Everybody there loves him, including the pastor, the harmonist, the choir girls and the boys. He runs errands at the church—he keeps the Bible ready, the song books, he even arranges the chairs. He likes doing that kind of work. He is affectionate towards everyone. Whenever a guest comes home, he will get them to sit and offer them water. He likes it when we have visitors.

Nimi: In the early years, when Aditya was about four, things were quite difficult, actually. But the good thing was that he was a happy child. He would smile a lot, laugh and play. He was a very naughty, happy child. Even though he was not toilet-trained and was quite hyper—he would run out on to the road—he was a happy, cheerful child. There were some things about him that we could enjoy. He used to behave in a very cute way many times. He loved to sleep with us in our bedroom and would wait just outside the door with his sheet, watching us all the time. The moment we said he could join us, the moment we gave him permission, he would leap into our bed! He always followed my instructions, listened to me more than he did anyone else. He understood my tone, my language, everything. So, I didn't really have a problem ... I have learnt that unconditional love is important. And children like Aditya love you back unconditionally. Theirs is a very pure sort of love and they do show care also, at least Aditya did. It isn't as though they take advantage of you. Sometimes I would be down with a migraine and Aditya would want something. He would pull me out of bed and take me to the kitchen and ask for it. Then he would take me back to bed and see that I am lying in the same position!

If there is one big regret that you have, what is it?[*]

Swati: When we moved to India after ten years in North America, it was just not the right time for Karun. Though he did show signs of recognising his Indianness, he had begun to think of himself as a Canadian. Karun still thinks of himself as Canadian. The move back to India has not quite worked for Karun. At the time, we were seeing the big picture. We were

---

[*] There were no responses from Waheeda and Joyce to this question.

really concerned about Pramath being happy professionally. He was afraid that the institute in Chennai where he now teaches would not be ready to wait another year. And I kept saying, 'Look, let's wait one more year. That way, at least some things will settle.' But Pramath was really worried. I don't know if one year would have solved all the problems, but at least some things could have got solved. Karun was about twelve at the time. He had just started having seizures and we had to stop one of his medications and then this other thing, this frightening thing—let me call it violent behaviour (though it is really not that)—had started. And we had no clue why. It was mind boggling. It seemed to just come out of the blue and was over before we knew it! Gone! No residue of it left! And we didn't know from where it would strike us. And then, just two months before we left, we got some very thorough blood work done for Karun, just because it was covered by insurance. And the results showed that he was acutely low in vitamin D. We bought a bottle of that but in the whole move back to India—which we did without much planning—it was like, okay, we have to go now, we just have to go now, just drop everything and run, pack up your things, sell this, throw that, put the rest in a cardboard box and we will see. It was like that. Then, of course, everything else in your life goes out the window, right? It was hard, under such circumstances, to maintain any kind of routine and we were barely able to keep up with the medication for Karun. The medication related to the seizures we maintained. But the vitamin D itself was lost somewhere in the ocean of madness. And then seeing a doctor here in Chennai was not easy. Plus, we had to live close to where Pramath worked, for I saw how long he would take to commute otherwise. That meant we were far away from everything and seeing a doctor was difficult. Back then, there was nothing in this neighbourhood. And in any case, Karun was not willing to enter hospitals or waiting rooms. We gave up and so he just lay there, curled up in bed in a fetal position for practically three whole years. And then we made our first trip to Canada and suddenly he was on such a massive emotional high that he overcame all those issues and we had a fantastic trip! But then we came back and he had a relapse!

Pramath: The most obvious mistake was returning to India in 2009. But then if we hadn't done that, we would have been in the US, which too was a mess. When we went to Canada from the US, we had to do a lot of things—fix up a school for Karun, find an apartment. Donna Winter (I still remember her name) actually offered us something else, which would have benefited Karun. ABA certainly, along with a lot more. But we went to a private school and paid for ABA. Just regular sensible intervention, small class sizes with a decent teacher-student ratio. I forget what. I wish we had taken that up. So does Swati. In the mornings there was this therapist from the behavioural institute whom we paid. Karun had been doing well in the university school in the US. Of course, we also had some ABA at home there. In fact, he got a lot of speech therapy. We would hire graduate students in speech and language from the university and they would do the therapy under the supervision of the speech therapist. Karun really flowered out there—he was speaking full sentences; he had a social life. He was there between the ages of three and four and a half. We should have pursued some of that in Canada. But the structure in Canada was different. There were other challenges too. So, there is a regret box in my head which I suppress. It comes out every few months. Right now, it is in suppressed mode. I have never been physically tough with Karun. But I lose it sometimes like any other father would.

Shoba: The mistake we made was that without telling anybody we pulled Diya out of Vidya Mandir and put her in another school. We did this because she was weak in math. We should have tackled that in a different way. The principal of Vidya Mandir later asked us why we did that. Apparently, they would have exempted her from math had we kept her on. The culture in the school we shifted her out to was not good.

Sankaravadivelu: Later, when we shifted her out to Ananya Learning Centre from this school, the principal of Vidya Mandir told us that they actually had a system whereby they referred children to Ananya and then took them back again when they were ready to re-enter the mainstream. We really should have kept her on at Vidya Mandir.

Shoba: And the CBSE board allows exemption from math in the case of some children. As parents, we get so anxious ...

Sankaravadivelu: That was the biggest mistake we made. It was a big, big mistake. A school like Vidya Mandir would have been so accommodative.

Shoba: It was a very inclusive school.

Sankaravadivelu: And they were all so fond of Diya. They also took a liking to Shoba because she had taken such good care of Diya and taught her so well. They asked her to join them as a teacher.

Shoba: I joined Vidya Mandir without any prior teaching experience! I didn't have to give a demo or anything. They just told me to join when Diya was in third grade. She was doing really well. At Ananya Learning Centre too, they really helped her.

Sankaravadivelu: Yes, but the only thing was that it was a sea change for her. It was a shock to her. She could not accept it. But one teacher there, Janaki, helped her a lot. She even went and stayed in her house for a couple of days. That lady too has a daughter who is adopted. The problem with that centre was that they had students from very diverse social and educational backgrounds. They were also very strict. They wanted to help. But the students there tended to be rebellious. Many do not enjoy much parental support. So, we had a tough time. But somehow Diya sailed through.

Shoba: Maybe we should have found out earlier about her hearing impairment. She did not utter a word … Even when we were told she could not hear, I said, 'No. She *can* hear. She is active. She turns …'

Sankaravadivelu: I think we would have done the same thing. If I were to start over, I would not have put her into that international school. That is the only thing I would have done differently. Otherwise, I think we went by the book. Even in Bala Vidyalaya, she was one of the few who could talk clearly.

Mamtha: I regret that I didn't take Tarak out as much as I ought to have. I made that mistake. We parents run around for physiotherapy, for occupational therapy, for speech therapy. Rarely, very rarely, do we spend time with the child in public places. I feel very guilty that I didn't do that. I feel I should have gotten him used to being in public places. Also, that way, people too grow used to children like him. If he had been habituated from that age itself, then we would have become used to it.

I used to see the rashes on his buttocks and think, 'Oh God, if he walks that alone is enough. How can I carry him around everywhere?' Once he walked, I thought he should speak. Mothers always think, 'What's next? What's next? What will my son learn?' We forget about these public places. We have to actually take them out. Now there is a greater degree of awareness because parents are taking children with autism to public places. But even then, it is only very young children who are taken out.

Nimi: Aditya was making steady progress till the age of thirteen or fourteen. There was a regression after we shifted from the apartments where we had been staying for many years. He was about fifteen then. There was also the puberty factor but the shift affected him a lot. In the old apartment, our neighbours had really started to accept him. They would talk to him. He used to cycle around the block and the boys were friendly with him. People would stop for Aditya when he was out cycling and he too was quite careful. The day we left that apartment, Aditya understood what we were doing. He was watching us pack. On the last day, the house was empty of furniture. We were leaving for T. Nagar. Aditya wouldn't budge! He just entered the house and said, 'No! No!' It was so sad to watch him that way. What followed was real regression, you know. The new apartment was in the heart of the city. There was no place for him to walk or cycle. So, Aditya took to just sitting on the sofa. It was scary. He even stopped walking properly. He started to walk sideways like a crab. He wouldn't go for his bath; he started wetting his pants. That was the most difficult time in my life, I think. He was so independent in so many ways before that. It was very, very difficult. That was when I decided to leave Aditya's father. I was forty-five that time and Aditya was seventeen. I was not able to do anything beyond that, you know. I had to start all over from giving him a bath. And Aditya had gotten into a shell, he was not communicating, he was not happy anymore. He became a very different child; a person. So then I thought, even if I leave his father, it is not going to make a difference. I felt very bad leaving him but I also knew there was no point; there was nothing I could do anymore.

Are you more accepting of your situation now? Have you come to terms with it in some ways? What do you want most for your child? What do you hope for?[*]

Swati: For us, there was this distraction of moving countries. I would make peace with things and then have to make peace all over again. Now, all I want is a retired life for all of us! That's all! That is the important thing. You don't need anything else.'

Pramath: What we want most for Karun is security, happiness … We have always wanted Karun to have a larger life than just us. A community which he understands, where he can share his joys and his grief.

Sankaravadivelu: We would like Diya to take up a job and work with 'normal' people in an environment that won't offer the kind of support as in school or even college. We are also concerned about her marriage. Will anyone accept her? That's a difficult thing. If I had a son and if someone were to ask me if I would consent to my son marrying a girl with a disability, I don't know if I would say yes. But there are examples. My friend's aunt is deaf and dumb. She has no formal education. But she is married to a man without any disabilities.

---

[*] There were no responses to this question from Waheeda, Joyce and Nimi.

Shoba: They have children, grandchildren. There's some hope at the end of this dark tunnel ...

Mamtha: I didn't worry too much about academics where Tarak was concerned. If he is given work in a hotel as a waiter, or if he is required to lift heavy weights somewhere, I think he will be a happy person because he likes movement. He is fine physically and can carry 10–15 kilograms weight. I feel he has to do some work, work that will make him happy; I am not concerned about the type of work. I am not sure if he will 'settle' or even how to define that 'settling'. Once he is in a safe place, and he is happy and has a good routine, maybe I would want to do something. Things will happen when they are meant to. So, I wait for that. But I still have that fire inside of me to help others. I think I was born to see Tarak grow and learn.

What would you tell other parents of children with disabilities, parents in similar situations?*

Pramath: Actually, we deal with that a lot. Sometimes it happens that we can see a child has challenges. Sometimes, a parent may even let us know that they have these worries. We tell them then that there are good chances that the child may have autism. Sometimes things turn out well and the child doesn't really have autism; sometimes they don't turn out so well. But when there is a diagnosis, what do I say? The first thing is this: for that parent, somebody has died. There is no point telling him or her these other things. These parents must understand that there is now a real child as opposed to the one they had imagined. There has to be a respectful period of mourning that you allow. When they reach out to me, I

---

* There were no responses to this question from Waheeda and Joyce.

say that this real child is as human and as wonderful as that other child, that there are things to look forward to, that his trajectory may be different but there *is* one. It is not a flat line—there are ups and downs, you need to be engaged with the child. I say to them, spend time with your child. One of the problems is that you can exhaust yourself running from one point to the other. Everybody knows something that you ought to be doing. Stick to one or two things, available nearby. You need to spend time with your child. In India, how do you access the second layer of services, somebody who can take your child out for a walk and so on? It is difficult. The school we sent him to in Chennai didn't work at all. When I would go to fetch him (it was a long commute), he would have his head down on the desk. If he spoke a word or two, they would say he was making progress. Sometimes, we would have just dropped him and on the way home, they would call and say you may have to pick him up because he is very agitated. This is bad for the child and for you. It is important to find communities of parents and kids right here. We can't subcontract things to somebody else. It is important for the kids to see people other than their own parents, even if it is canned and contrived. All I am trying to do right now is to take Karun out for long walks, to try to engage him. I think the most important thing is that the focus should be on the child, not on yourself or on other things such as your career.

Swati: I don't know how useful this story is to others. I would like to say to other parents, 'Accept your children as they are, even as you work towards making them better and stronger. Children have to be delighted in.'

Shoba: I would tell them that there's hope. Early intervention is the best for the child. Even we were late. We acted on it as soon as we realised and she started talking …

Sankaravadivelu: If the parents are in a remote village, how can they come to Chennai? But we tell them, if you want to educate your children, if you want to get them to talk, bring them to a school like Bala Vidyalaya. Nowadays, many opt for cochlear implants. We consulted a famous ENT for Diya too. He told us very clearly that she didn't need an implant. She was fine with a hearing aid. Her progress has been exemplary, she is good enough. Only children who cannot cope with hearing aids need a cochlear implant. Even children with implants have to undergo training in order to talk. But they can hear sounds much better than Diya can. Minute sounds, like birds chirping, she cannot hear. Even with the best of hearing aids, she can't hear these sounds. I would tell parents, take them to Bala Vidyalaya or other such places, get them to talk, there is life for these kids.

Shoba: I would advise them to visit the ENT regularly, to upgrade their child's hearing aids.

Mamtha: At Vidya Sagar, I observed that there are different kinds of parents, parents who have it harder than we do. Some of them are also financially worse off. So, instead of dropping Tarak and coming home, I decided to volunteer at Vidya Sagar. He was in the day centre. Vidya Sagar allows parents to accompany their children until they turn four or four and a half. This is during the period of early intervention. After this period, parents are required to leave the child alone. It was then that I decided to volunteer. I decided to help other parents. I remember this child called Manikandan. He was from a slum and had multiple disabilities. He only had auditory abilities. So, I thought I could help out by feeding him. Whenever I cooked variety rice, I used to pack one box for him and made sure he always had healthy food. I always kept thinking of ways I could be of help. Even though I was going through a tough time myself, I always had that thought at the back of my mind.

Nimi: It is an emotional thing, parenting a child with a disability. I always believed that your feelings—your worries, your sadness—are transmitted to the child. If you manage to stay calm, that will definitely help the child. Consistency in training is important. It is very difficult but you should also be prepared for nothing happening. You have to just accept it. We see two types of mothers or parents in general—one lot have totally given up; they have no hope but they still take the child for therapy or whatever though they are so sad and bewildered, and then there's the other lot who somehow or the other want their children to get better and end up demanding too much of the children, who then become very aggressive. I also feel we should teach these children basic life skills first. Academics and so on come only much later.

Lessons in Walking from Zach

Kelli J. Gavin

Kelli J. Gavin of Carver, Minnesota, is a writer and professional organiser who focuses on home and life organisation. She has over four hundred pieces published in over fifty publications. *I Regret Nothing: A Collection of Poetry and Prose* and *My Name is Zach: A Teenage Perspective on Autism* were both released in 2019. She blogs at www.kellijgavin.blogspot.com. Her social media handles are: @kellijgavin on Facebook, Instagram and Twitter, and @keltotheg on TikTok.

Josh and I were married in 1995. I am a professional organiser of events, a writer and a public speaker. We have two amazing kids—Zach, who is seventeen, and Lily, who is thirteen. Zach has autism. He is able to speak and have his needs met. He enjoys life, is funny, kind and artistic. He loves to swim, golf and spend time with friends. Lily is goofy, outgoing and spunky. She loves music, playing outdoors, riding her bike and acting in plays. We live a very calm and structured life. We try not to do too much in a day, as that is what works best for Zach and for the rest of us. Zach thrives on knowing what the day ahead looks like. He enjoys days that allow for time to play.

As many parents of special needs children know, the difference between a successful day and a day filled with chaos and tears is really all about being adequately prepared, planning out the day and then sticking to the plan. By tears, I mean parent tears. The child's tears are usually a given. Digressing even slightly from the anticipated structure of the day can cause meltdowns for Zach. It can result in emotional upheavals and an inability to reclaim a joy-filled day.

When Zach struggles with sensory overload, he needs to just take a step away. Away from the upset, the memory of what has gone wrong or not as planned. He needs to walk, sometimes for long distances. Until his mind stills, until his heart returns to an even pace. He needs to listen to the birds and hopefully meet a dog or two along the way. Our walks are special. It is usually just Zach and I. Zach's observations in nature, his keen sense of hearing, his amazing mind and conversation can often restore even the weariest of souls.

I have learnt many simple lessons from my son. Always walk when you can. Country dirt roads are usually the most fun. Explore, and never be afraid to get a little lost. Sticks and corn husks make cool makeshift dolls. Dogs are better one at a time. Be very quiet when approaching creeks and springs; you can often hear the frogs. Always stop to admire the green grass that matches the green barn. Remember to sit under the big old pine tree. The pine cones can be used to make funny faces. When all else fails, just walk. Walk. Until your heart calms, until your breathing returns to a more measured pace. Walk the dirt roads until you feel as if you have walked enough.

Then turn around and return. Return to friends, return to family. Return to the green grass and the green barn. Smile as you see the bright red barn through the trees. Walk back across the bridge over the creek slowly and enjoy the sound of hollow footsteps. Just take time away. Time away from the busyness of life when just the sound of the birds talking and the breeze blowing are the most important things to focus on. Where the clouds are breathtaking and the grasshoppers are giants. Just breathe.

Zach finds walks restorative, where the calm he so desires is not only found but cherished. As Zach's smile returns, he is able to interact with me and even show me more of what he enjoys. His intentional eye contact and laughter is contagious with each new singing bird. When Zach's line of sight follows a scampering squirrel or unknown rustling in the trees, my attention is drawn to the beauty of our surroundings. Zach understands that sometimes the calm is all he needs to seek. The destination isn't something to concern himself with. Zach's example of being present in the moment is an example I learn from, daily.

I have found that our lives are so much simpler than the lives of friends. Our days often revolve around outings to thrift stores and garage sales. Garage sales actually take up a large amount of our time. There is joy found in a spiral-bound notebook, a *Blue's Clues* bright orange VHS tape, small Dora toys from the free bin. Music is always appreciated. Thank you for playing it during our garage sale adventures. Great pleasure can be found under the shade of an expanse of trees. We love running our fingers through the long green grass as the warm breeze rustles the leaves above.

Most of our outings just involve casual walking. From the car to a new adventure to a garage, to a new shop, to a park that beckons us for a new experience—but walking is what each day produces. Walking and discovering new sights and sounds, sometimes of unknown origin. My own anxious heart is calmed and shifts away from the busyness of life after these walks with my son. All because I take the time to relax and see the world through the eyes of my special seventeen-year-old.

This Kind of Child

K. Srilata

I distinctly remember that bleak November day in 2013, the skies grey and grieving just as I was for my daughter whom we had pulled out of school a couple of months ago. There she lay huddled under a light quilt, unmindful of the blare of school bus horns, seemingly oblivious to the life that was passing her by. I grieved because I was convinced that she would never find her way back into the maze that counted as 'education'. It seemed to me that she was lost, and hopelessly so. If the liberal Montessori school to which we had admitted her could fail her so badly, what chance did she have in any other? And, by extension, what chance really did she have in this difficult world? She had joined India's millions of 'left behind' children and it didn't seem to me at the time that she would ever 'catch up' with the rest. Dyslexia (or whatever it was that passed for it) had felled her. It had tripped her up. As I sat at her bedside that morning, it occurred to me that my daughter had no place to turn to, that the four of us—her father, her brother, her grandmother and I—would *somehow* have to become that place. Home was the only school that would take her.

My daughter was nine when we took her out of school. I couldn't help thinking of her first day at school. She had gone in with sparkling eyes and feet that danced to music that only she could hear. My husband's aunt remarked once that she was like a small butterfly—with her light and happy movements. All through those early school years, I had read to her and to my son stories and poems at bedtime and whenever the opportunity presented itself. My son became an independent reader at some point. This transition had been so smooth, so organic that I barely noticed. As for my daughter, she clearly enjoyed listening to the stories I read her and knew them all by heart. She had a great sense of the spoken word, often spoke in metaphors herself and had sound literary judgement. Except that reading (and writing) did not come to her easily.

By the time she turned seven, I was quite certain that something was amiss, that there was a reason why Ananya wasn't getting around to reading even though she was obviously bright and curious, open to new ideas and was possessed of a burning desire to learn. And she was certainly no lazier than the average child. I urged her to read books meant for early readers (with large type text and plenty of pictures) but she turned away from them. It was almost as though the sight of words made her *physically* ill. Her struggles in school too began around this time. The Montessori school she was in transitioned its students almost overnight from a system of sensory and activity-based learning to reading, writing and pen-paper tests. Her butterfly-self vanished and a heavy grey dullness settled over her, a dullness I found alarming. More and more, it became clear to me that there was a clear *mismatch* between my daughter's intellectual abilities and her ability to process text, something I was soon to learn was a classic symptom of dyslexia, which is one aspect of what is now called Specific Learning Disability (SLD).

In the October of 2009, on the advice of a friend, my husband and I took my daughter who, at the time, was still in school, to Nirmala Pandit. Nirmala (who is featured in this book) was a special educator and also the founder of the Madras Dyslexic Association (MDA) and one of the kindest, most warm-hearted of people I have had the good fortune to meet. She was, at the time, living in a large independent house and so to my daughter it felt as if we were just visiting someone we knew. Nirmala related to us not as someone who was an 'expert' in special education and therefore was the last word on it but as someone who was genuinely interested in the child and open to exploring along with us the ways in which she could be helped to learn. She put us instantly at ease, listened patiently as we narrated our woes, and then ran a few simple assessments on Ananya. A few days later, we received her neatly typed up and detailed report which ended with the lines:

Ananya has dyslexic kinds of difficulties in the areas of spelling and writing. This must be attended to immediately. The variation in her performance and apparent short attention span are related to this difficulty. She does not have any difficulty in attention and memory. It was a pleasure to meet and to work with Ananya.

So finally, we had an explanation of sorts, a name for what Ananya was struggling with. This cut both ways, of course. It helped to have that explanation, to rest knowing that Ananya's issues were caused neither due to laziness nor due to a general lack of intellect. But the labelling was a fraught, difficult thing. After all, much of the time, she was a child, not a dyslexic child, not a child with a specific learning disability. And that is how we related to her, that is how we wished the world would relate to her. The United Nations Convention on the Rights of Persons with Disabilities came to the conclusion that it is when a person who has a certain condition interacts or comes into contact with attitudinal or environmental barriers that a 'disability' is created. We know this as the social model of disability, a model that has challenged in a fundamental way the manner in which we think of disability. In my daughter's case, and in the case of millions of other children with dyslexia, it is school and its ideological trappings that constitute the biggest 'attitudinal and environmental barriers'. Schools are set up in such a way that these children are bound to fall through the cracks. A vicious cycle of failure that comes at a huge psychological cost is the inevitable result. For children like my daughter whose dyslexia was 'mild', it is often impossible to be certified as dyslexic, to be eligible for any reasonable accommodations. Sometimes, the only choice—especially if you want to remain within the school system—is to stay under the radar, to offer other excuses to explain your 'poor' performance in tests and exams or go along with the unfair remarks often made by class teachers and principals, remarks attributing the child's poor performance to her laziness or inattentiveness in class. All this and more happened to my daughter when she returned to the school system in grade eight after over a year and a half of being homeschooled, but that is a story for another time.

Our meeting with Nirmala Pandit also meant that we now had to begin to *do* things and at the time, we were staring at the lack of a clear path. It was overwhelming, like all 'diagnosis' tends to be. There was grief of course, grief at all that Ananya had already suffered, and the suffering that a hidden or invisible disability such as hers would bring in the future. We were aware that the diagnosis meant she would probably not have the happy, carefree childhood that others her age enjoyed. She would have to work harder than her peers just to get by. Nirmala had told us that early intervention was key and so we knew that we had no time to lose. We had to break our grief down into actionable units. We could not let ourselves be destroyed by it.

A few days after the reports came in, I went back to meet

Nirmala, this time on my own. She suggested that I put Ananya through the 'remediation' that was required. She felt I would be able to manage the teaching that this entailed and lent me resource materials and books. Overnight, I acquired a new role: that of special educator. I had been asked suddenly to man a truck when I hadn't the foggiest idea how to drive an 800; the truck was full of precious cargo and I had to arrive at my destination with everything intact. What I remember most from those years is how my body felt—the crashing fatigue, the physicality of my heartache. As for what Ananya must have gone through, it hurts me to even imagine it. She would return wiped out from a school where the teachers did not get her. And there I would be waiting to teach her spelling rules and the idiosyncratic exceptions of English, after a long day spent lecturing at my day job. We would settle down—the two of us—after a quick snack for there was 'no time to lose', not with the kind of school systems we were up against. Ananya was sometimes reluctant to learn. She would turn sullen and uncooperative. Often, despite my resolve to the contrary, I would become impatient with her. Which, of course, made her all the more sullen and uncooperative. Teaching Ananya made me both less and more of a mother. She came to depend heavily on me and I on her dependence. Tantrums, frustration, apologies and making up were part of the territory. I remember one evening sitting there and watching Ananya pierce with the sharp edge of a pencil the sheet of paper on which she was supposed to be practising her writing. I remember worrying if one day she would pierce her own skin with the same degree of violence. I remember the guilt I felt each time I lost my cool with her. For I knew very well that none of this was her fault. That is how the cards had been dealt. And she was precious cargo that I had to deliver safely. I hadn't a choice. We hadn't a choice. She was making progress, yes. But it was far slower than what school would allow for. And sometimes, just when it felt like some things were falling into place, she would begin to flounder and we would have to begin all over again. She was way behind her peers, despite working on her reading and writing skills every evening. One day she asked me, 'How did Ani learn to spell? Did you teach him these rules as well?' I hadn't the heart to tell her that her brother had never had to learn spelling rules and exceptions, that life had handed it all to him on a platter. I often worried about my son for, at this point, my daughter needed all my attention. I wondered what he made of it all, whether he felt neglected. I felt helpless. But there was nothing to be done. My husband too got into the role of remediator—he taught Ananya maths, which was another area of difficulty—not because of any conceptual issues but because Ananya often switched or misread numbers and had difficulty with sequencing. As for the spectre of second language which, in her case, was Hindi, it proved to be her undoing. It was cruel to expect someone who was struggling to decode one script, to also decode another, altogether different one. We took Ananya to MDA for a more formal assessment, hoping that they would recommend her exemption from Hindi. After a three-hour long assessment process, the MDA handed us a report which, while acknowledging that Ananya had a 'cumulative history of dyslexic features in the area of spelling and writing' and that her skills in Hindi were 'below class level', went on to state that an exemption from Hindi could be considered after a review the following year. The MDA also recommended that we put Ananya through some occupational therapy in order to fine tune her fine motor skills. We took Ananya for a few

sessions in occupational therapy. The lady who worked with
Ananya was stern, though not entirely unpleasant. I am not
sure to what extent these sessions helped, but there it was.
We shared Nirmala's reports as well as these reports from
the MDA with the school, but of course an exemption from
Hindi was out of question. Ananya's teachers were mildly
sympathetic and not unkind. But the system remained blind
to her struggles, to her failing self-esteem. School was nothing
short of an obstacle race. Ananya would work really hard and
end up with abysmally low scores on her test papers. She
ended up fearing the teacher's red pen more than anything
else in her life. I remember switching to blue when I graded
my own students' papers. School was mountains of work as
far as Ananya was concerned. There was simply no getting
around that. I hoped that all this hard work would only pay
off in the long run. It wasn't going to reflect on her test
scores that year or the next or even the year after. In fact, it
soon became apparent that the best we could hope for was
a pass grade. But how do you expect a child to square this
all? When the only 'reward' that schools offer are by way of
grades, how does one persuade a child to work despite the
absence of rewards? Especially when that work is completely
invisible to her teachers from whom she expects a certain
validation, teachers who assume she is being lazy or difficult.
The trouble with dyslexia is that it is invisible. It is what
people think of as a relatively 'easy' or 'small' disability, a
disability that isn't as hard as other more obvious, visible ones.
Dyslexia is that small but incredibly sharp and painful thorn
that has lodged itself in your foot and hurts you when you
try to walk. It is a thorn that no one ever sees. It trips you up
when you least expect it, make you feel small and stupid. The
indignities of constant 'failure' and the mistaken assumptions

that the person is just not working hard enough, or is just too stupid to get things right can take a huge psychological toll. During one particularly fraught round of first term exams for which Ananya had slowly and painstakingly plowed her way through *Around the World in Eighty Days*, she ended up failing the English exam. It was then that the decision to pull her out of school was taken. Ananya did not hesitate for a single moment when we asked her if she would like to be taught at home. My son, struck by the unfairness of what she was going through, declared that it was high time she quit school. Ananya was clearly miserable at school—this, despite the fact that she had a few friends she was very fond of. On friendship day, Ananya would return from school with her wrists and arms covered in friendship bands. She would have spent the night before painstakingly crafting friendship bands to gift her friends. When she left school, these friends would phone every single day to ask when she was coming back. She is in touch with them to this day. Leaving school must have felt like an amputation—the loss of friends and their company, the loss of an entire ecosystem.

After a short break in Goa, we decided to plunge in a Pollyanish way into full-time homeschooling, a beast we had little idea about. I set about doing the homework for that and learnt that there was a small but growing body of homeschoolers (and even 'unschoolers') in India, especially in cities like Pune and Bengaluru. Unfortunately, there weren't too many homeschoolers in Chennai. I discovered that people homeschooled their children for a variety of reasons. Some did so for religious reasons. Others because their children were struggling or were far too 'bright' to be constrained by schools. And some others because they did not see the point of school at all—they felt it wasn't worth it—the stress and

the pressure of school all for the sake of a piece of paper at
the end of twelve long years or more. These parents taught
their children informally at home and typically signed them up
for the NIOS (National Institute for Open Schooling) exams
when the latter were old enough to take them. This way they
would still end up with a certificate that was recognised by
most colleges in India, including the IITs. It was a brilliant
way of cutting through the crap. The unschoolers were the
most quirky of the lot, for they did not believe in teaching
their children in any formal way. Nor did they see the need for
any kind of certification. Ananya and I attended a conference
organised by a homeschoolers group called Swashikshan,
in Khandala. Entire families turned up for this conference
and it had the feel of a picnic. On the whole, it was a most
remarkable experience. Ananya made a few friends too. The
conference reversed traditional hierarchies by placing children
on panels. I remember listening to a sixteen-year-old boy
who spoke of his repeated failures in school and how he had
quit school and registered for the NIOS but had ended up
failing those exams as well. He said that his repeated failures
had taught him a lot. It had taught him, for instance, how
to be a good teacher. He was now tutoring other children,
helping them with the NIOS exams. For the first time, I was
meeting people who didn't think of school as an inevitability.
They didn't seem in the least anxious about the fact that
their children were not in school, that they were 'footloose
and fancy free'. In fact, if anything, they seemed to be proud
of this fact. It occurred to me that opting out of the school
system is the single biggest act of resistance there is in modern
society. For when you opt out of school, you automatically
opt out of so many other societally organised ways of being,
including certain kinds of working lives. Of course, there was

also this issue of who has the 'luxury' of opting out of school altogether, and then what about the millions of children in a developing country such as India whose parents would kill to get them into a 'good' school? This was also the time when the Right to Education bill was introduced. This complicated the lives of homeschoolers, for their children were 'out of school' and the state was making efforts to recruit children into the school system. At around this time, the NIOS system withdrew its grade eight level certification which meant that homeschooled children would receive their first official certification only when they were old enough to be in grade ten. Until then, their status was liminal, nebulous. This was equally true of children who attended non-formal schools (schools that were not affiliated to any particular board). So many of these children were happy as they were. They were not 'deprived' in any way. They had access to a different kind of an education altogether. To force them to go to school would not have served any purpose.

In his book *Deschooling Society*, Ivan Illich takes what is arguably an extreme view of schooling. He argues that students are schooled to 'confuse teaching with learning, grade advancement with education, a diploma with competence, and fluency with the ability to say something new'. Illich argues that not just education but also society as a whole would benefit from deschooling:

Everywhere the hidden curriculum of schooling initiates the citizen to the myth that bureaucracies guided by scientific knowledge are efficient and benevolent. Everywhere this same curriculum instills in the pupil the myth that increased production will provide a better life. And everywhere it develops the habit of self-defeating consumption of services and alienating production, the tolerance for institutional dependence, and the recognition of institutional rankings. The hidden curriculum of school does all this in spite of contrary efforts undertaken by teachers and no matter what ideology prevails.

We homeschooled Ananya for a year and a half. Since both my husband and I worked, we took turns taking her along with us. On one day of the week, she stayed home with my mother. My husband was in charge of teaching her math and science, while I continued to work with her on English and also did some social science with her. There was, of course, a lot of juggling involved—given that both of us worked and that we also had another child and parents who needed our attention from time to time. On some days, I was convinced that we were doing the right thing. It was clear to us that academically at least, Ananya was making great progress. She started reading very fluently and during one particular month, we found that she had read close to twenty books! Her writing improved as well, though spellings were still something of a challenge. So, things were most certainly looking up. School-stress and pressure were no longer factors. Our bodies, for one thing, were far more relaxed. Just to liven things up, we gave our home school a name—Flame Learning Centre. At the end of the academic year, I even created a 'formal' report of her progress and Ananya was thrilled. One thing that sustained Ananya right through these years was music. Ananya was a singer and was training in pop and Western music. More recently, she told me that back then when things had been rough, music had come to her rescue in a way that nothing else had. Her own incipient interest in music therapy as a way to heal psychological pain and trauma dates back to these years. If music was Ananya's coping strategy, mine was long conversations with other mothers whose children had difficulties—not just Ananya's kind of difficulties but other kinds of difficulties because of which none of the solutions on offer in the mainstream worked. I soon realised that these conversations during which sometimes we traded dark jokes and, occasionally, some imperfect 'solutions' based on joyous loopholes in the system, were hugely useful. Those conversations were comforting. They taught me that there were ways and ways of being a parent. There we were—a small, motley group of ship-wrecked parents, stranded, with our children, on a remote island. The only people we could turn to were each other. There did not appear to be any rescue boats in sight. All the other parents were safe and dry on the mainland. It was this situation that partly prompted the writing of this book.

To return to my narrative: at some point, I chanced upon a learning centre for homeschooled children in Chennai and enrolled Ananya there. It promised a certain degree of flexibility and openness that we liked, and gave Ananya a place to go to during the day and the chance to meet other children (though all the children there were far younger than her—the only one who was about her age left soon after she joined). Here, Ananya received some external validation perhaps for the first time in her life. She learnt some elementary weaving and dyeing. She went through a phase where she was knitting and using the 'rainbow loom' obsessively.

The decision to put Ananya back in school was taken for a variety of reasons. We were beginning to feel that she was missing out on so much socially, that she felt, maybe, a wee bit lonely despite the fact that she was going to the learning centre almost every day. It was also getting harder for us to homeschool her, given pressures at work. Scheduling things and just navigating the day was getting to be increasingly difficult. We were also reasonably confident that Ananya would now manage to stay afloat in school, not struggle as much as she had in the past. But most importantly, Ananya too felt she was ready to have a go at school again.

Securing admission into a school though was far harder than we had bargained for, though we ought to have anticipated that. For one thing, it is nearly impossible to get a child admitted into grade 8 (which was the grade Ananya was age-wise eligible for) in most schools in Chennai. There are simply no vacancies. What made it harder was the fact that Ananya was out of school. It wasn't a case of transferring her out of one school and into another. We applied to another 'liberal' Montessori school affiliated to the Cambridge board, having heard good reports about it. I spoke to the principal, explained Ananya's background and even shared all the reports we had. She assured me that the school was an inclusive one and I took her at her word. Ananya took a test in maths and English. The next day, we got a call from the school. They asked us to come and to bring Ananya with us. At this point, we felt quite sure that they were going to give her admission. But what followed was the stuff of nightmares. The principal asked my husband and I to go in, while Ananya waited outside. She held out Ananya's answer sheets, pointed to all the 'errors' and asked us how they could possibly admit 'this kind of child'. That phrase went through my heart like a stake. I remember coming out of the principal's office in a state of shock. I remember Ananya asking us in a low, gentle voice—'So have I gotten in?' I remember telling her that I would explain it all to her later. I remember her falling asleep in the car on the way home. And I remember weeping quietly over that betrayal, that accumulation of small insults. I remember, too, the sympathetic look on the face of Kasi, whom we had recently employed to drive us. He told me later that the school must have wanted a donation from us. I have often wondered if his theory was right but have no way of knowing, of course. We knocked on the doors of some other schools as well, with no luck. In the meantime, a small school had opened up in our neighbourhood. The school had applied for affiliation to the CBSE and were admitting students. A neighbour of mine who taught there suggested that we try our luck there. So, I went to meet the principal, taking Ananya along, armed with various craft and art pieces that she had created during her homeschooled years. The principal was a simple man. He was clearly not very comfortable in English. The school he ran was not an 'alternative' school. And yet, I realised at once that he was a man to whom children really mattered. He listened as I told him the whole story, asked Ananya a few questions, looked at the scarf she had woven and remarked, 'Each child has his or her own talents. There's no problem at all. She can join class 8 straightaway, maybe take French as her second language. My son struggled with Hindi but found French easy.' So that was how Ananya became a school-going child again. Thanks to the simple, easy kindness and good sense of one man.

To our delight, she blossomed in that school. At least this was how it appeared to my husband and I, for Ananya confided later that she had some rough times with a couple of her classmates when she got to grade ten. The school was fairly mainstream in its pedagogy and approach, but the fact that there was a clear structure and a relatively small class ratio appeared to help. The choice of French (over Hindi) as a second language helped too, just as the principal had predicted. Ananya didn't have to worry about decoding two different sorts of scripts—the Roman would do. Even though Ananya was never top of the class academically, she won the hearts of her teachers (especially that of her wonderfully kind class teacher) and of her fellow-students. She went on to become school pupil leader and sports captain. She was elected to the former position. And she did this all in the quietest, gentlest way possible—by just being herself. I look back often to those years and think of just how far human kindness can take us, what it can enable.

Ananya spent three years in that school. During this time, she began to talk of wanting to pursue psychology later in college. The school was planning to start a humanities group for grades 11 and 12 but unfortunately, because of its relatively small size, dropped the idea. In the meantime, Ananya took her first public exams—the tenth grade boards—and, to our joy, not only did she survive them but also fared well. She had to be switched out of this school and into a new one because of her stated intention to pursue psychology. The new school was about as mainstream as it gets, with a population of 15,000 odd children. It was driven by a results-culture and was clearly biased in favour of children who test well. We had been through the entire gamut—from homeschooling to a high-pressure school environment in which Ananya often said she felt like a 'speck'. The transition wasn't easy on her. In fact, frequent and difficult transitions are often a price that children who are wired differently pay in the absence of systemic support in regular schools. But familiar as she was with the challenges of school transitions, Ananya displayed a remarkable resilience. Recently, she declared in a dour, wise old-aunt sort of way that school 'has never been a happy place' as far as she is concerned.

At the time of writing this, Ananya is on the cusp of another transition—this time from school to college and adulthood. The story is far from over. I am aware that the time has come for us to encourage her to find her own way, even though for my husband and I it has become a lifetime habit of support, advocacy and occasionally rescue where Ananya is concerned.

We will, I am sure, face new challenges, acquire new learnings, make some mistakes, fall down a lot. But that old thorn in my daughter's foot isn't as sharp as it once used to be. It doesn't prick us as much. It doesn't trip Ananya over as often as it once used to, and when it does, she is better prepared for it.

Over the years, what has struck me about Ananya is her ability not just to survive but also to thrive even in the most difficult of environments. It has become more and more clear to me that she has decided to let that label go, that she does not identify as one. In her own story, the story that inaugurates the book, the word 'dyslexia' makes its appearance only once. More and more I am beginning to see that it is the environment that creates and exacerbates disabilities—a fact that holds true for all the people in this book who are its protagonists.

BOOK FIVE

Siblings and Children

Note

Of all the disability stories we hear, it is the stories of siblings and children of people with disabilities that remain the most invisible. Stories of the ones who are sometimes drawn into care work and emotional labour, pressed into service by families stretched to the limit. Stories of quiet presence, of difficult responsibilities assumed lightly, of adulting, of learning to love, of letting go of the self, of watching from the sidelines the struggles of a brother or a sister, the sadness of being that witness, the things one learns from it.

The Ship of Life: *Nanak Naam Jahaz Hai, Chade So Uttre Paar*

Sarabjeet Dhody Natesan

Sarabjeet is an associate professor of economics at Krea University. She lives in Chennai with her family. She is currently working on her first book of life memories.

Biji's house was big and had a place for every conceivable thing or activity: a drawing room, a dining room, bedrooms, storeroom, first floor, balconies, terraces and even a room converted into a gurudwara. However, in one corner of the big house, and to me the most important corner, was a bed on which lay a man. At first, this man seemed to be the most important man in the world, or perhaps the laziest man ever. All he had to do was call and someone would come running. He was carried wherever he had to go, was hand-fed on the bed and everyone who visited my grandmother's house sat in only this room—the big house was not used at all. Bit by bit, as I became physically conscious of the life in that big house, I was struck by the dim light, by the heavy curtains on the only road-facing single window on the ground floor, that too on the backstreet. The house was recessed from the street, and the moat of a verandah kept all conversations and sounds and sights and sighs inside. And all the sounds and sighs of this man, Bawa, were unheard too by the outside world. He made it really easy for this to happen, because his voice, even when he was upset and angry, was never more than a raspy whisper, and did not even reach the person whom it was intended for.

As I soon understood, Bawa was not an important person. Neither was he lazy. He would often ask me to get him a drink of water. Not only did I have to get him a drink of water, I also had to slowly pour it into his mouth and wait as he drank it. I was my father's water girl too, and would hand him the glass and be off, but when it came to Bawa, I had to fetch the glass and after making sure that I did not accidentally cause him to choke on the water, take the glass back into the kitchen as well. This was something I never did for my father. It annoyed me no end, for it got in the way of my very inquisitive ways, my desire to find where everything in the big house was kept. I didn't understand why the man couldn't rise from his bed and fetch his own glass of water. Nobody spoke about it, it always hung in the air, and eventually, I too, like the rest, put together the jigsaw pieces of the man on the bed, realising that Bawa was never going to walk, or even move.

This man was my mama, my mother's younger brother. As a child, travelling from a violently fractured country to his new home, Bawa was afflicted by a mysterious illness. Nobody knew where it came from. It started as a fever and slowly debilitated him, leaving him paralysed from the neck down. I was too young to understand much of this, but once I knew, I no longer grudged being his water and glass carrier.

As I grew older, it struck me how I had never really noticed my bedridden uncle and his confined life. It was so natural to find him there, being helped to sit, eat and exist. He read a lot, listened to the radio, watched television diligently and wrote a lot of letters—well, made *us* write letters *for* him. All of us were supposed to read his mail to him, write his replies and talk to him about our lives. It kept him going. There was never any pity; we did nothing out of pity or duty. He was there and he asked us to do things for him and we did them.

Bawa's bed was in the biggest room in the house, right opposite to the kitchen, next to the window. In a dormitory-like setting, about three feet away was his youngest brother Param's bed and next to that my grandmother's double bed. It was on this bed, next to her, that I would sleep, whenever I stayed overnight. This arrangement was so that if Bawa needed any help at night, there were people around to help him. My grandfather slept in the next room; he was old and not well enough to be of much use. Barring my nana, the other three men in the house were my mamas, my mother's younger brothers.

Every morning and evening Biji would do a prakash, a required ritual of opening the Guru Granth Sahib and reading from it.* Gurudwaras, as far as I was concerned, were fun places—the karah prasad, the langar, the beautiful, mellifluous shabads, all enough to put me in a good frame of mind. But even with a gurudwara in her house, Biji seemed sad. Even when she smiled, I never saw the sorrow leave her face. In fact, the big room of the big house seemed sad. Until I became old enough to know the difference between happiness and sadness, to understand pain and loss, I tried everything to make Bawa and Biji happy. I stood on the window ledge of their big room, singing songs, giving speeches, acting in imaginary dramas, but like the sad princess from the fairytale, who never laughed, my grandmother too never laughed.

Bawa, however, did try to enjoy my visits and would constantly ask me questions about my school, my friends and

---

* This is what is required by the tenets of Sikhism. The Guru Granth Sahib has to be opened and read from every day. It is a living entity.

about the outside world. Whatever my inadequate observation of the outside world and my irritation at being prevented from doing other things would allow, I would answer and run.

Later, when I understood more, I too saw much to be sad about. My Biji's life seemed a contrast of extremes, a life of abundance and a life of emptiness: one son confined to bed since 1949, paralysed from the neck down; another son, Arjan, a victim of a tragic train accident, which took away one limb from the knee down; her husband, who had lost his hearing and memory and would go missing, wandering off. Her sadness was like a mountain; you could see it, feel it, touch it and you could climb it as much as a couple of hours' visit would allow. We did climb it, sense her misery, and at the appointed hour of our departure, let the stone roll back down the slope, only to see it return to the top of the slope on our next visit. Only my mother seemed to carry pieces of her mother's mountain back home with her.

Once I understood this, I also understood my mother's frequent visits, her unspoken concern for her mother and her need to sit with her and share her grief and anguish.

After doctors gave up on Bawa and nothing seemed to work, the family, though highly educated and professional, turned to the only source known to all in times of trouble— religion. Gurudwaras were visited, akhand paths (non-stop reading of the Guru Granth Sahib) were organised, holy dips in the gurudwara sarovars (water tanks) and chalias (forty days non-stop visits to the gurudwara, come what may) were undertaken. Unfortunately, religion too failed them, just as everything else had.

Transporting the wasted body of a young man was not easy and was done with the help of another young man, Bawa's younger brother, Param. Param became the sole physical caregiver to Bawa, who refused to let strange hands touch him. Anointed caregiver without consent, Param also became responsible for his wandering father, Sardar Gurdeep Singh; his older handicapped brother, Arjan, who too needed emotional support, and his mother, Sardarni Raj Kaur, whose sadness was apparent to everyone. He was there for everyone, for everything and every occasion. He was there to buy rations, to get vegetables, to get train tickets organised, to arrange pick-up and drops, to cook in case Biji was not well, to attend weddings and funerals. He became the face of the family. In the midst of it all, he managed his career as a handwriting forensic expert. And in the bargain, he became good at hiding his own sadness.

Their lives—Bawa's and Param's—were an exercise in ritual. Bawa had to be woken up early. He had time set aside for his personal care and at that time, we were not allowed into the big room. Despite his condition, he lived within the tenets of Sikhism—his long hair was unshorn, and during his weekly bath, he ensured that his hair was washed as well. He was given a clean-up and his clothes were changed every day before Param left for work.

The big house which was constructed after the family moved there was built on two floors, yet no one lived on the top floor. Param was on call downstairs and Arjan was unable to climb up. The garage had been converted into an office and this is where Arjan and Param would meet their clients (both being in the same profession). The handwriting and forensic work was started by my agile grandfather when he had entered India. And it was easy for his sons to follow in his footsteps and take over the business. The area under the stairs had been converted into a darkroom to process photographs and evidence from property documents, wills and other *kanooni dastavez* (legal documents). There was a huge demand for their work as a newly partitioned India came to grips with wills and property transfers and individual shares in joint-family properties. On days when Param's work took him to small courthouses in Delhi and Uttar Pradesh to give evidence for clients, Bawa's daily requirements had to be taken care of before he left. Biji and Arjan managed the rest as the day progressed. But Bawa would be on pins and needles till Param returned. With no cellphones—not even very many fixed line telephones—his and my grandmother's eyes would be always on the clock. Bawa knew Param's train schedule by heart and would calculate the exact time of his arrival, factoring in the time it would take his brother to get off the train and walk home. The train station, a stark reminder of one tragedy in their life, thus remained an important part of everyone's days.

With doctors and their science, and even religion struck off the list, the task of finding a cure for Bawa's ailment was placed in the hands of faith-healers. Someone only had to mention in passing that a miracle had been performed—a blind man who was suddenly able to see, or a man in a wheelchair who was now able to walk or, really, anything along those lines—and my father would arrange for a car and a driver dutifully. Biji, my mother and Param would be deployed to accompany Bawa to visit the healers, who often operated in far-flung rural areas. Nobody complained of the trouble or the stress—not Bawa, who had to sit in an Ambassador car with a backbone that refused to comply with orders to be straight, nor the group, lovingly calling itself a *jatha* (a religious group) on a quest.

These missions too would fail. They would return, crestfallen and disappointed, without a cure in hand. With nothing to fall back on, Bawa would go into a state of deep silence. He wouldn't speak to anyone. He would ask Param to turn him over, so that he faced the window, the curtains drawn close, and stare sadly, silent tears rolling down his face. We knew that this was his time to not be disturbed. With little other understanding, this was what we would do and leave him alone.

Occasionally, Bawa would ask me to rearrange his papers, his postcards and his letters. His memory was phenomenal. He would tell me to take the third postcard from the bottom, written on a specific date by a specific person and keep it aside because he had to respond to it. My sister's handwriting being clean, precise and firm, that task was left to her. Mine was to organise and prepare Bawa's correspondence. The letters were all about the magical cure that he was looking for. It was a cure that he was not to find till the end of his life, but his quest was unending, as was his hope, which rekindled after every discouraging episode. I think it was this hope that kept him going, through the slow atrophy of his body, his laborious breathing.

At some point, Arjan's wife, Aagya Kaur, was added to the legion of caregivers. The other siblings married and left, their paths their own. Nobody had the time, the ability or the determination required to keep the show going. It was a job that was open to all, yet one that fell on the lives of a few. And these few had accepted it without knowing what it was all about. Later, when they had fully comprehended the enormity of the job, they carried on with a sense of resigned duty.

Bawa was required to eat his meals sitting up. At mealtimes, he was gently hauled up by Param. Biji would then fold his legs under him in a criss-cross position. He would then be made to lean forward, his elbows resting on the chowki. This way, he did not have to be propped up. His meals were served on a plate and kept on the same chowki, and he was fed one morsel at a time, very patiently. When you feed a child, you know that soon enough this will end, for a child does not have to be hand-fed forever. But with Bawa, it was unending—three times a day, seven days a week, twelve months a year, without a break, for as long as there was life in that body. Param did the heavy lifting and Biji or Arjan the feeding, for Aagya had taken over the kitchen by then. Bawa displayed occasional bursts of temper, more at the unfairness of life than at the way he was taken care of. Sometimes, it seemed as if his anger was directed at everything and everyone. Param would often visit our house, his elder sister's. It was his getaway, his time to be pampered. My mother would run us around to get cold drinks and pakoras the moment she saw his Vespa enter the front gate.

Life was not easy for Bawa, and his sadness sometimes enveloped the house. On those days, my grandmother would ask my mother to come and spend time with her. As always, like a little foot soldier, I would accompany my mother. While they spoke, I would wander around, open almirahs and drawers in the room upstairs, play with Blackie, a big black pet dog, drink sweet tea and play in the big garden outside.

As children, visiting our grandparents' home was still the best outing that we could have. There was a big house, a beautiful new mami who loved us and food and treats for asking. There was a separate drawing room where the television set was kept. The Sunday movie at our Biji's house was a weekly treat. We would all get together there, and Param would carry Bawa to the room and prop him up on a big comfortable chair. The kitchen was in the next room so dinner was an easy-going affair. While Param fed a seated Bawa, we would all go to Aagya mami and get our customary ghee-drenched chappati and a bowl of daal. A tastier meal cannot be imagined. On the days the Hindi movie was a repeat telecast, we spent the evening in Bawa's room, chatting and talking. He would lie there quietly, listening and smiling, just satisfied that we were all there and that he was not left out, forgotten. Our sense of ownership over these childhood privileges was complete.

It came to me later that other lives too had been sacrificed to the endless demands of caregiving. One such life was that of Aagya mami, Arjan's wife. That young and blushing bride who came seeking the life of her dreams had been saddled instead with responsibilities she was not prepared for. Only my father noticed this and said so. But his admonitions were often drowned in the perpetual silent sorrow of the house. Aagya mami did what she had to do unflinchingly and without expectations. She just blended into that house of needs.

Param's marriage had also been sacrificed at the very same altar. His beautiful and educated wife led an unfulfilled life, with her husband always at the beck and call of his brothers. Their need for him had always been greater and their demands too pressing for him to refuse. After a particularly painful fight between him and his wife, my parents had been called in to mediate. A deafening silence had fallen over the house when someone asked how a marriage could survive if all Param had the time for was his disabled brother. Param wiped the tears from his eyes and said, quietly, 'He is my brother, my life and my kirat (commitment).' And with those words, he turned on his heel and walked away.

Biji, with her worry-lined and tired eyes, too upset to question Waheguru and her faith, continued to do a prakash every day. After the customary reading of the Granth, she would come downstairs and recite a few lines of the gurbani to Bawa. Till the end, her faith held her together. If ever Bawa, overwhelmed by sadness, told her that he wanted to end it all, be gone from this body of his, she would turn to him and say, '*Oh Bawaya, mere bahche, Nanak Naam Jahaz Hai, Chare So Uttare Paar* (Says Nanak, remember the name of the Benevolent One, meditate on it; whoever boards the ship of life will be dropped at its final destination).'

He Was Mine to Look After

An Interview with V.R. Krishnan

V.R. Krishnan is a retired officer from the Life Insurance
Corporation. His brother, Narasimhan, has Down's syndrome.
Krishnan and his wife are Narasimhan's primary caregivers.

Srilata: Let us begin by talking about your ages—yours and
your brother Narasimhan's—and what your earliest memories
are of him.

Krishnan: Narasimhan is sixty-four years old and I am
seventy-three. He is physically healthy, although he does
struggle with problems associated with his condition, such
as constipation and loss of vision to the tune of 80 to 85 per
cent (in both the eyes). His mental retardation was assessed
around twenty-five years ago and was about 82 per cent.
Now, I am sure it is a lot more.

The earliest memories I have are those of Narasimhan's
childhood, when he was around two, and I, eleven. At that
time, there was hardly any awareness about mental retardation.
There was just a broad term for children with Down's
syndrome and they were called Mongol children (this, of
course, owing to the false perception that they shared facial
similarities with the Mongolian race). Why, we had not even
heard of the term 'Down's syndrome'!

Although he was two years old, Narasimhan was not even
able to turn on his side. He would just lie down until someone
turned him over. His head was not erect and slanted a bit,
and saliva constantly dripped from his mouth. So, naturally,
my parents began to seriously wonder if all this was normal

for his age. A doctor who examined him told us that it was a blessing that he did not suffer from hydrocephaly (water accumulation in the head) as well.

Srilata: Do you remember the time when his challenges and difficulties began? What was the diagnosis? When was he formally diagnosed?

Krishnan: The fact that he was not a normal child was a point of profound grief. We realised that despite being over two, he was unable to indicate natural instincts like hunger. For instance, he would not even cry for milk and would eat or drink only when food was given to him. It is all too easy to imagine the rest.

One of the first physicians to examine him was Dr A. Behannen. We were in Bangalore at the time. She confirmed that he had Down's syndrome. This was in 1957. We moved to Thanjavur the following year and then, later, settled down in Chennai, primarily because we could consult the renowned neurologists Dr Ramamurthy and Dr Kalyanaraman there. Amma and Appa also took him to Dr Saradha Menon, the famous psychiatrist at Kilpauk Mental Hospital. The prognosis for Narasimhan was unanimous: he would have to be under the care of someone throughout his lifetime.

Srilata: How did your parents respond to Narasimhan's challenges? What sort of therapies did they try? Did any of this work?

Krishnan: Quite naturally, my parents were very upset. Two things bothered them a great deal. The birth of a child with a disability was a burden to the family, primarily because they were quite old when they had him. Appa was then fifty-five and Amma, forty-three. Narasimhan was the eighth child, the youngest living child amongst all of us. Had our parents been younger, they might have been in a better position to personally care for him. They may not have had more children either. The second aspect that haunted them was the inevitable question of who would care for him after their lifetime.

Back in the 1950s, there were no therapists who could guide us on the rearing of such children. There were no suitable medications. I remember there was one tablet of Glutamic acid, called Nuerogluton, which was regularly given to him.

That is how Narasimhan's journey began. He was not able to attend regular schools, and special schools for children with disabilities were unheard of. My parents initially made arrangements for a private teacher. He was taught the alphabet and simple words in English and Tamil. By the time he was ten years old, we realised that the classes were not really helping. His comprehension had deteriorated and we had to discontinue them.

To improve his language and communication, all of us at home would constantly talk to him and engage him in various errands. We took care that he did not overeat and was always neatly dressed. We got him used to a normal routine and gave him simple household chores to perform. This way, he was reasonably fit. But this too lasted only for some time, for his ability to comprehend, process and react began declining rapidly.

Srilata: As a child, what did you make of Narasimhan's condition? Did your parents ask you to look after him? Did you feel a sense of duty even as a child?

Krishnan: The new arrival in the family, when I was just nine or so, was a thing of joy. He was very fair, soft like a rose, almost like a toy to play with. As his state of self-helplessness gradually grew, all of us siblings said that we would always be there to support him at all times and at all costs. What we forgot is that life causes one to embrace his or her own family, and siblings naturally take a backseat.

In a middle-class family like mine, the expectation is that the eldest son will take over the family reins when he comes of age. There was no necessity at all for this fact to be explicitly stated, for I was the eldest child. And since Narasimhan was also an occupant of the chariot whose reins were spontaneously handed over to me, he was mine to look after. He was not the only one. My third sister, Padmasani, who also suffered health issues like juvenile diabetes (this was without any family history), was determined to be with me, and chose to remain unmarried. She pursued her calling as a teacher but unfortunately died when she was just thirty-four. It was a big blow to the family. From thereon, with Narasimhan, it was an automatic transfer of guardianship. Moreover, since he was with me since his birth, I was bestowed with the duty of caregiver right from my childhood. There were a lot of compromises I had to make, which I shall narrate elsewhere.

Srilata: Tell me about Narasimhan's challenges at present. Has he gotten better in some ways? Is there a decline?

Krishnan: The challenges are many, but they are more for others than for him. You see, he is not in a position to understand what those challenges are. For well over two decades now, his capacity to understand and act accordingly has deteriorated quite fast and has reached a stage where we believe that no further decline is possible. I have learnt that mental retardation is a highly debilitating condition and that, depending on the severity, those affected become increasingly dependent on their caregivers.

Narasimhan does not know when he is hungry. He shouts on very rare occasions. He usually considers the corner of his room as the toilet. On very rare occasions, he goes to the toilet on his own but those times are few and far between. He just does not understand the concept of a diaper and it serves the purpose of nothing but an undergarment.

He is able to recognise no one except me, and me only as someone who takes care of him—not as Anna (elder brother), the term he used to address me earlier. It is only because he is familiar with this house that he is able to move about here freely. If he falls down accidentally, he is not in a position to get up on his own. Somehow, I have always intuitively known when something goes wrong and, thankfully, have invariably proved to be right. I have always been around to help him overcome any difficulty. As far as possible, perhaps because of our sheer experience and God's will, my wife and I are able to foresee things and act appropriately.

Srilata: How do you care for Narasimhan on a day-to-day basis?

Krishnan: You know, I have often joked that he should actually be living in the USA, because his circadian rhythm functions accordingly. He is asleep for most part of the day, and my wife and I find it difficult to keep him awake. Every day, my first chore in the morning is to visit his room to see his condition. He is usually sitting on his bed. For a newcomer or visitor to the house, it appears as though he is in a vacant or pensive mood.

We then guide him to brush his teeth—he has virtually none remaining—and then give him a glass of milk. He tends to get restless unless he is given a bath soon. Once that is done, he is usually calm. He eats his breakfast by 9 or so, after

which he just rests. We have to pull him out of his room at
1.30 for his lunch. He usually eats breakfast and lunch on
his own. Sometimes, we have to feed him. He has a cup of
milk in the evening and eats dinner by 8.30 every day. You
must remember that he has no recollection of time, so it is
entirely up to us to keep track and attend to him periodically.

In between, one has to take him to the toilet four or
five times a day. If we forget, there is the additional job of
cleaning the room as well! Occasionally, this also happens,
defying our constant vigil. Our going out of station is as rare
a phenomenon as a hen with teeth. On the few occasions that
I do have to go out of Chennai, my son, Badri, takes over my
duties. Once in a blue moon, in case my wife and I have to
necessarily go out of town for two or three days, my brother
Raghavan and his wife come and stay with Narasimhan.

Srilata: Your wife and your children have also helped take
care of Narasimhan. Can you tell me about that? Have your
siblings pitched in as well?

Krishnan: The greatest gift in my life is my wife. In my
younger days, whenever there was talk of marriage, I was
straightforward in telling those who met us with proposals
about Narasimhan, and that he would be with me throughout
his life. Many of them did not come back with the promised
alliance. I had the good fortune of getting Rukmani as my life
partner. I got married when Narasimhan was in his twenties.
He would never let anyone enter our private room. When my
daughter and son were born, he used to take care of them,
keep the feeding bottle to their mouths and untiringly swing
the thuli (cradle-cloth) till they fell asleep. My children have
been brought up alongside him and, therefore, have a very
soft corner for him. My elder sisters were married within

three years of his birth and their contribution after he was grown up was limited. However, my youngest sister, Vaidehi, was with us for a long time and so helped us care for him. Even after her marriage, she has always helped by coming and staying with us during emergencies, so that she can care for Narasimhan. Even now, when needed, she and her son visit our house and take care of him for a few hours. More recently, we have simply decided not to leave him and travel out of town.

Srilata: Have Narasimhan's struggles changed the way you think about life?

Krishnan: The knowledge that his everyday existence depends totally on me has made me think that there is no point in taking life too seriously. I follow the dictum 'prudence is the better part of valour' and live a life without risks, for I cannot afford to upset the family status quo in any way. Had it been only Narasimhan, perhaps he could have been managed even if I had moved out of this city and taken up a job elsewhere. However, given that I was responsible for looking after my aged parents, I simply could not think of it. Being a staunch Vaishnavite, I believe completely in karma. Even in my younger days, I knew that you will get what you are destined to.

I often recollect this verse from the Gita:

Karmanye vadhikaraste Ma Phaleshu Kadachana |
Ma Karmaphalaheturbhurma Te Sangostvakarmani ||

Your right is to perform your duty, but never for the results. Sincere and loyal work automatically begets valuable results. Never be motivated by the results of your actions, neither should you be attached to not performing your prescribed duties.

I should admit that this approach of mine has only brought positive results in both my professional and personal life.

Srilata: What impact has the presence of Narasimhan had on your life, especially in terms of your career, your marriage, your leisure time and your other responsibilities? How did your life change after the death of your mother?

Krishnan: In the early years of my job-hunting phase, I faced a lot of issues. I was an untrained teacher in a school in T. Nagar for about a year. The school correspondent was very happy with my work and offered me a job on the condition that I enrol for the one-year B.Ed. programme. He offered to pay the fees for the course as well. But how was the family to bear the loss of my salary for one year? I had to turn that offer down. In more than 90 per cent of my job interviews, I had to decline the postings if they were not in Chennai. This was much to the frustration of my well-wishers, for they often helped by arranging interviews for me. Before joining LIC, I worked in the income tax department for a few years and some private companies before that. Thanks be to the Almighty, for I was never wanting of a job even for a day.

I successfully completed several competitive exams for bank probationary officers but the out-of-Chennai postings stood in my way. At LIC, remaining in Chennai was an option as long as you didn't apply for a promotion. This was the perfect choice for me. I decided to take things as they come and play them by the ear. One of the significant moments during this time was my meeting Shri L. Khan, who understood my circumstances and paved the way for me to stay on in Chennai. His help moulded my professional career to a great extent.

Marriage was a great blessing in my life. I am grateful to have been blessed with such an understanding wife. Looking back on this journey, I am proud to say that during the forty-four years that we have been married, we have had no rift of any kind. We are the apple of each other's eye.

When everything in life is viewed as a duty, responsibilities automatically follow. Both of us believe that we are doing our duty and never do we think that we are sacrificing something. Thinking so would only lead to swollen heads.

We have our leisure time, albeit in a limited way. We do not expect anything and, therefore, we don't feel let down by any turn of events.

My mother's death did not make a significant impact on Narasimhan. But for us, the sadness of losing a person to guide us and remind us of the most important things, and of priorities, still lingers.

Srilata: What has been the most difficult part of being Narasimhan's primary caregiver?

Krishnan: I have had the opportunity to study a report on the lives of parents of both mentally and physically handicapped children. The challenges mentioned in the report indicate high levels of stress in families with handicapped children. However, despite this, families have been able to find successful coping strategies. I am of the opinion that this is 'auto generated'—in families where the nurturing of a child with mental retardation is viewed as a burden, self-induced stress and negative impact heightens. If the situation is accepted realistically, the positive impact enables them to stand by the child.

Narasimhan cannot take care of himself and requires assistance and constant care in every aspect. So, my work as his primary caregiver encompasses just about every duty.

Srilata: What things about Narasimhan have brought you happiness?

Krishnan: Fortunately, our parents consciously ensured the disciplinary upbringing of Narasimhan. He was not allowed to excessively indulge in food, clothes or anything else. Therefore, listening to what we say and following instructions has become his habit, quite unlike a child with mental retardation (MR). Even as a child, his daily routine was strictly adhered to, and today, this has saved us from several challenges that caregivers of adults with MR typically face. He has no health issues, except truncated growth. Senescence in MR adults (gradual deterioration in physical and mental state) is generally rapid. However, we have not found this in him. He doesn't look his age. It is the absence of body-mind coordination that poses all the problems. Normal health issues, like cold and fever, do not affect him much. Even if something happens, he somehow becomes alright without any medicine. As I am getting old, I am unable to decide whether this is a boon or bane.

Srilata: What sort of social support do you wish for so that people who have the same challenges that Narasimhan does can have a better life? What kind of support would *you* wish for as his primary caregiver?

Krishnan: There is a lot of awareness now. And yet, we do not have the time and energy to take enough care of disabled people in our own families and so, we start looking for the assistance of trained people. We think our responsibility ends there. Actually, it begins there. We must monitor progress to know if we are on the right track. We must spend a good amount of time with the afflicted. Regular physical contact like hugging and showing our concern through words and facial expressions makes them happy and instils confidence in them. Also, attending special courses on how to cope with the retarded and afflicted is greatly useful. Both parents must involve themselves in the upbringing and make other siblings also understand the problems of the afflicted child.

Nowadays, the symptoms of Down's syndrome are detected in the early months of pregnancy. Parents have the option of MTP (medical termination of pregnancy). If the child is born, the earlier the support system is started, the better. Special schools must be contacted and the child should be able to go to a nurturing environment. Constant attention and care is of paramount importance so that the child is instilled with confidence. Generally, children with MR are known for their stubborn attitude and that must be addressed from the early stages of childhood. The general tendency of parents is to pamper the child, considering the disability. However, this is not in the child's interest.

Children with such disabilities will show interest in some activities and these must be identified. The plus point with such children is that they are not easily distracted once they start doing an activity.

They very easily become emotional and resort to violent behaviour when their wish is denied. Patience is the only way to deal with it. Otherwise, violence will become a habit.

Srilata: What, according to you, are Narasimhan's biggest strengths?

Krishnan: He has no undue desire to eat or overeat. He will listen to even my grandchildren and doesn't behave harshly with them.

Srilata: Did you feel at any point that your parents paid more attention to Narasimhan than they did to you or your other siblings? Did you resent that, even mildly?

Krishnan: The fact is that it was we siblings who paid more attention to him. Our parents had their own priorities. Ours was a large family with frequent visitors. Besides, he was the youngest child, so there was no such feeling that he was being given more attention than the rest.

Srilata: What do you worry about most of all when it comes to Narasimhan?

Krishnan: Times are such that the present generation has no spare time and they work under a lot of stress and strain. Even if they sincerely desire to help anyone, they are not able to. So, my earnest prayer is that the duty of being caregiver for Narasimhan should not become a nuncupative legacy to my son or daughter. I am confident that he will have a decent exit during my lifetime.

This One Purpose

A Conversation with Chetna

Chetna is the sister of Tarak, a young man with DAMP syndrome. She is currently pursuing her masters in speech and language pathology.

Srilata: Tell me about yourself. How old were you were when Tarak was born? What was your life like before his birth? What was it like after?

Chetna: I am currently pursuing my masters at Ramchandra Medical College and am in my final year. I have chosen a field called speech and language pathology, basically a paramedical field. The main reason I chose this field to specialise in is my brother, Tarak. My mum wanted me to purse a bachelors in commerce—a popular choice with most Jain girls. But watching the last speech therapist that Tarak went to—her name is Zainab—I was sure that this is what I wanted to pursue. I am twenty-three years old now and Tarak is nineteen, running twenty. He was born on 1 January 2001. I don't recall much of the years before he was born. All I remember is being around my parents a lot. I remember my parents telling me that I had just had a baby brother, that he was going to come home from the hospital. When Tarak was very young, my parents realised that he was not walking. He would just move around on his butt. So, a friend of my father's or someone known to him advised him to take Tarak to the beach, dig a pit in the sand and place him neck-deep inside it. Everyone was focused on his muscular development and strength. My parents would lock me in the house every morning as I lay asleep and take him to the beach to try out that remedy. I remember waking up one morning, realising I was alone and not being sure of what was happening. There was a bell tied to the grill. I kept banging on the door, waiting for my parents to return.

We used to do quite a lot in those days. We used to travel quite a bit. Sometimes, a friend of ours—a photographer—would come by and take pictures of Tarak, of his things, of all the places he had been to. This was to improve his communication. I found it all very exciting. I never hid anything from my friends; they knew about Tarak. When I look back, that was one of the best things I chose to do, because people tend to hide these things. I don't get the point of that at all. Tarak is very active and social. When you meet him for the first time, he will talk to you as though he has known you for a while. People say that he has features of autism. But contrary to the characteristics of autism, he is actually very sociable. One day, I had my friends over. Tarak approached one of them and tried to communicate with her. He held her wrist and perhaps because it was the first time she was seeing someone like that, she got really scared. That picture is still fresh in my mind. Even though that girl was, and continues to be, my best friend, this memory haunts me. As Tarak grew older, things became difficult. My cousins would plan trips and outings but would hesitate to invite me. This was because I would not go anywhere without Tarak. It was very immature of me perhaps. But I have accepted this state of affairs now—not a 100 per cent but may be 90 per cent! I do go out with my cousins sometimes, because I know now that there are places to which Tarak cannot go. If I feel that we can take him some place, we do take him.

Srilata: Tell me about your parents. How did they respond to Tarak's challenges?

Chetna: My mum got married when she was nineteen. She was born and brought up here in Chennai, though she is a Jain. My dad is from Rajasthan. His family migrated to Chennai to run a business. My mum was very bold. Or that's what I have heard from her sisters—my aunts. As a child, she would manage her schoolwork, her accounts and the shop. My grandfather had a medical shop. She would sit at the shop and help, she would cook ... Then she got married. She was twenty when I was born. When Tarak was born, my mum was twenty-three. So, until Tarak's birth, I guess we had a very normal life. We were just like any other family with a newborn. My father has a clothes store. He sells children's clothes. So, he would get me dresses and they would dress me up. I have some pictures of that. After Tarak was born, everything came to rest on my mother's shoulders. I won't blame my dad. He was completely preoccupied with his business. I am not sure how he really felt about things. Was he not accepting of Tarak? Was he confused? Didn't he realise the severity of the issue? I'm not sure. My mother would break down every now and then but she was determined to make Tarak better no matter what. I credit all the progress Tarak has made till date to her. I remember her telling me that she used to carry Tarak in her arms, all the while holding on to my little finger as she talked to doctors. This was so she could figure out what was happening with Tarak. Till Tarak was eight months old, he appeared perfectly normal, except that he would cry continuously and no one knew why. If he touched a hot object, apparently he wouldn't draw his hand back. His milestones were delayed. These were the reasons why my mother had to literally go from doctor to doctor. But not one of them told her Tarak's was a lifelong condition! The doctors diagnosed the condition quite early but nobody told my mother that this was not something that could be cured, that Tarak wasn't ever going to develop in the normal ways. They told her instead that Tarak would be a very active person, that he would get into an engineering programme or become an athlete because he had so much energy. That's what all the doctors told her. Had they told her that Tarak would always have issues, my mother would have been prepared.

It was only when my mother took him to Vidya Sagar[*] that she got a clear picture. At Vidya Sagar, they counselled the family. That's when my mother realised that Tarak's issues needed much more of her time and energy than she had anticipated. So, he started attending sessions at the early intervention centre at Vidya Sagar right from the age of eleven months. He continued to be at Vidya Sagar until he turned eleven. He was given physiotherapy, speech therapy and occupational therapy, and my mother would work with him at home all evening. She also worked at Vidya Sagar for seven years. Tarak and she would leave home in the morning and return only in the evening. I never got much time to spend with my mother because she spent all her time with him. Tarak now goes to a small centre called Edkadaksha Learning Centre. He is there from 10 a.m. to 3 p.m. My mum doesn't accompany him. He goes there by himself in an auto. We have trained him to keep quiet. The moment he comes back home, my mum has to be there.

My mother talks to and counsels parents of children with special needs. She invites them home, puts them in touch with a network of people who can help. She's very meticulous.

---

[*] Spastic Society of India, Chennai

Srilata: Did you resent this as a child?

Chetna: If I did, I don't really remember. Maybe I never gave it a thought. And not thinking really must have saved me back then! But nowadays I think a lot. And that thinking is what gets me into so much trouble—with my health and so on. Back then, I just accepted life as it was. I moved to a different school only after class ten. I had a lot of Jain friends. I would watch them go out on weekends, do whatever they wanted to. I didn't have that choice! These small things would hurt a lot. I would question it a lot but there were no answers. That was just the way it was. Since my parents, my mother especially, was so exhausted, I couldn't just go where I wanted to or do what I wanted to. My father is an amazing person. His actions speak for him. He discontinued his studies back in Rajasthan and came down to Chennai to pursue his business. Given his background, it must have been a challenge for him to accept Tarak's condition. My dad realised at some point that Tarak was not going to be able to take up the family business. He spent a lot of time getting the house organised for him, making it safe for him. Everything in this house is organised keeping Tarak in mind—the height of the terrace walls and all of that.

Srilata: Tell me about your relationship with your brother. Is it a typical sibling relationship at some level?

Chetna: It is just like any other brother-sister relationship. But the manner in which we communicate with each other is different. I can't talk to Tarak just as you would to a normal sibling. But I do get mad at him and he at me! When he hits me or hurts me in some way, he tends to forget it at once. That is perhaps due to his condition.

But at the same time, he knows that what he has done

is wrong and he will admit it in his own way. I don't think normal siblings do that. There's a certain honesty to him, a child-like quality.

Srilata: Are people in your neighbourhood supportive and understanding of your situation?

Chetna: For seventeen years, we lived in a rented house in Royapettah. My father got this house constructed for the sake of Tarak. At Royapettah, we faced a lot of trouble from the house-owner because of Tarak's behaviour—his screaming, and so on. My dad often says, 'I don't mind even sleeping on the floor but I had to get a house of my own for the sake of Tarak.' Since we own this house, we don't really have to worry. But even now, we have issues with our neighbours. We tried making friendships. It's been only three years since we moved here. There are so many children living down this street and there is an association. So, we thought it would be a good place for Tarak. Every evening, we would have five or six children over at home. If it was a weekend, then we would have more—ten or twelve. My mum would cook for all of them, play with them, just because Tarak wanted friends. But after a point of time, parents started telling their children that if they came to our place, they would become like Tarak. The children actually stopped coming. It was all very disturbing. Tarak is a boy who is into routine. He is fixated on it. Though he didn't understand the concept of time, come evening he wanted his friends to visit. When everybody suddenly stopped coming, we had a tough time managing him. There was no way for us to explain these things to him. It was very difficult but we managed it and then we held a group meeting on the street. I told my mum to speak. Only then did people understand. But these days we don't encourage anybody to visit us on a daily basis. We have now prepared Tarak. We have told him that people may visit and spend some time with him but that they will also be going back.

Sometimes we feel it is all too much, that this is never going to get better. But on the other hand, if Tarak hadn't entered our lives, we would be just like everybody else. Life would never have a bigger purpose. The three of us—my mum, my dad and I—have this one purpose. As I have already told you, my father is not very educated and is a complete introvert. But if he gets to know that one of his customers has a family member with a disability, he promptly shares my mother's number with them and tells them that she will be able to help them. We have never been ashamed of sharing our story with anyone, especially if it's going to make somebody else's life even a little better.

Srilata: What do you think will enable Tarak and others like him to have a better life? What sort of support do you dream of in an ideal world?

Chetna: In an ideal world, people would just mind their own business. It is unnecessary for people to comment on Tarak. Some days ago, we took him to a temple. We were unable to get a cab on the way back and my mum decided that we would take Tarak back home by bus, because he really likes to travel by bus. We waited for a long time at the bus stop. Fifteen minutes into the wait, Tarak lost his temper. He has no tolerance for waiting. We finally got him into a bus that was not very crowded. Tarak sat down but one of the things he does on buses is to keep moving. He likes to get off at every stop and so on. When my mother told him to stay seated, he lost his temper and let out a loud scream. So, everyone, right from the driver to the passengers, *every single person* turned and looked at us. I know this is only to be expected. But my point is that in any society, you are going to have different sorts of people—all five fingers of our hand are not alike. There are two things I don't want: I don't want people to show sympathy and I don't want people to label Tarak in any way. People with disabilities should be treated just the same as the others. It is hard to care for a person who has difficulties. Life can be a real struggle. We may have visitors but they come and go. Nobody knows or understands our real struggles, the day-to-day struggles. At some point, you begin to wonder, what sort of life is this, because you have to face these issues every single day. It isn't as though it is ever done. And on some days, we face really huge challenges.

Srilata: What sort of future do you visualise for Tarak? For yourself?

Chetna: Actually, I'm blank about this. I don't know what awaits. My parents feel that I should get married and settle down in life. Until recently, I felt that I should only marry someone who will help and support Tarak. But my mother (with whom I fight a lot) explained to me that while it would be great if I found such a person, I ought not keep this in mind as a pre-condition. But I do know that I will be there for Tarak—out of love. I'm really interested in psychology and I also like doing a bit of photography. I also write. Once, when my mum fell sick, I took care of Tarak. I wrote about it on this app called Wattpad. So many people ended up reading my article. Writing has given me a name, an avenue. It has allowed me to vent my anger, describe my happiness and pain.

That Letter Grade on the Report Card

Aniruddha Kambhampati

Aniruddha Kambhampati has an undergraduate degree in law from O.P. Jindal University. He is currently pursuing an LLM at the University of Cambridge, UK. The quickest way to his heart is talking cricket or Harry Potter.

Perhaps the very first thing I noticed about my sister Ananya were her eyebrows. This might have had to do with the fact that there was a cute little mole positioned close to one of them that I found fascinating. Another early memory is the way she would clamber on to my bed (her feet were so tiny!) so we could play a board game together. Actually, I am not quite sure if this was actually a board game—or even whether there was a bed in that room back then—but this is how I remember it. Apart from these hazy recollections, what I remember about Ananya is the fact that she acted really hyper around us family and grew totally docile around other people.

When Ananya began to experience academic difficulties at school, I assumed, at first, that this was because she wasn't putting any effort into her schoolwork and that she was always looking for an excuse to get away from it. Somehow, I wasn't able to empathise with her mental state and maybe I never fully will. Perhaps one has to go through what she has in order to be completely empathetic. It didn't help either that I had just around that time moved to a school which believed that achieving academic excellence and all that crap was just a matter of will.

When my parents decided to pull her out of school and

homeschool her, I remember not being quite convinced by their decision. I felt that this would rob her of the experience of school life—the friends and the memories you make. I don't think I could (at that time) look at it all from a purely academic point of view, given that for me academics was secondary to everything else about school life. In hindsight, I feel convinced that homeschooling Ananya was the right choice at that time. I think she desperately needed a breather from the toxic environment she was in, so she could gradually regain some confidence and understand that it was okay not to be book-smart. In my opinion, the duration of her homeschooling—a year—was *just* right.

Witnessing Ananya's struggles with the school system has meant that I have stopped thinking of school from the perspective of the majority. These days, I judge a school on the basis of how those on the margins—those from other states and minority religions, those with disabilities, those with different learning styles, those who are not fluent in the medium of instruction, those who fail in almost every paper, those who are not in the least 'popular' or extroverted—experience it. A school should be a place that caters to the needs of every child, a place children feel happy to go to, not a place they are glad to get away from.

Having Ananya for a sister has meant that I have become more critical of the teaching methods employed by schools. My hatred of harsh teachers has definitely intensified. Schools should stop glorifying those who score well on exams and demoralising those who don't. I really wish they would change the way they test students, that is, if they feel they have to test them in the first place. I believe teachers should be open to re-teaching a class if required. They should grade students for the creative ways in which they have responded to a particular topic or question, conduct oral exams and even encourage students to pick their preferred mode of assessment. I don't think any of this is hard to implement. It is just a matter of will.

Watching Ananya's struggles has also made me see that a fundamental duty of any school is to teach its students about disability, mental health and discrimination on the basis of gender, caste, race and class. I think these are matters that have been completely brushed under the carpet by the schooling system in India (certainly by the CBSE system) and that is a shame. For if there is anything in the world that you ought to learn as a six year old, it is a basic sense of humanity. My sister is compassionate, friendly and creative, but none of this was valued by the school system.

Though a major part of my schooling was in a conservative school where all that mattered was the letter grade on your report card, growing up with Ananya has taught me that there is always more to a person than meets the eye; that intelligence should not be measured against a singular axis.

My Brother's Vanishing Act

Vanshika

By day, Vanshika edits academic manuscripts on neuroscience and medicine. At night, she turns to her pen and writes of her muses, the foremost being her journey as a sibling to an individual with Down's syndrome.

My mother paused, took a deep breath and wondered: Should she beam at me for uttering my very first words, or act on the bombshell I had just dropped on her? After all, my eleven-year-old brother with Down's syndrome was known for his frequent vanishing acts! He was a mischievous kid and made sure to hold our attention and to keep us all on our toes. She had to take a split-second decision.

The spark in my brother's grin remains fresh in my memory to this day. Twenty-five long years haven't succeeded in erasing the charm he exuded in every move he made, everything he said.

As the sibling of a child with Down's syndrome, I have a lot of untold stories. After all, I breathed, sensed and experienced a world completely different from that of most others. My mother tells me with both a spark and pain in her eyes, how when she was pregnant with me she would gently place her hand over her womb and say, 'Hey baby, there's a very special guy waiting for you out here. Take good care of him when you come.'

No wonder the first words that spilled out of my mouth were what they were. 'Mumma, bhaiyaa gaya.' Mom, my brother has vanished.

Twenty-one years later, he has vanished, claimed by death. And we had moved heaven and earth to make sure he would live on for just a few more days than his medical condition would allow. We played tug of war with death.

I recall, to this day, the time I used to spend at the special school he attended. I would silently watch him and his lovely aura as he went about spreading love and joy to those around him.

Wrapping his arms around his mates, he would announce with pride: '*Yeh Mashu hai—mera bhai.* (This is my brother.)' He would then glance at me with pure, unadulterated affection. I was only six at the time but I knew even then that my journey with him would not be an ordinary one.

I am not sure what it was that prompted my brother to cast me in the role of his brother, what prompted him to refer to me not by my given name—Vanshu—but as Mashu. Perhaps it was because he observed how fiercely I guarded him in every potentially threatening social situation that made him feel uneasy. In all those twenty-one years, not one Rakshabandhan would go by without him tying a rakhi on my wrist, upturning convention altogether. He didn't care what the world thought. And he instilled the same courage in me.

My brother's presence shaped my thoughts and my perspective on life. I am who I am because of him. He spent his days sketching his impressions of the world, painting the walls of our home if he felt like it. Who can stand in the way of an artist? I am lucky for I got to be around him, to witness his life. I got to be the person he loved most in this world. I got to be his bhai, his Mashu.

When it comes to the parents of a child with special needs, most people display sympathy and compassion. But when they meet that child's sibling, they usually say, 'Oh, I am sorry, you must feel as though all the attention of your parents and family is focused on your brother.' Which is far from the truth. What I want to tell people is this: My brother parented me better than my own parents did sometimes, offering me the gentle love of a mother and the fierce protection of a father. And as for that parental attention which you say he received more of than me, I was more than happy about it.

Be it the piano lessons I brought home for my brother to learn along with me (because the tutor told us point-blank that she could not figure how to deliver these lessons to a child with special needs) or the academics I helped him with (something that his special school was blind to), my brother's life was tied to mine. I lost myself in him.

'*Mashu, mai tumse bahut, bahut pyaar karta hun* (Mashu, I love you very, very much),' he would say every day. This, even when he was in hospital amidst a sea of doctors and nurses poking him with needles, even when he was hooked to his dialysis machine.

After he passed away, Rama maasi's words pierced my grieving heart and gave me strength: '*Beta, Guddu jahan bhi hai, woh kabhi tujhe akela nahi chodega. Tu jab bhi use man se yaad karegi, woh tere paas hoga. Ise hone se koi nahi rok sakta, koi bhi nahi* (Wherever Guddu is, he will never abandon you. Whenever you think of him, he will come to you. No one can stop this from happening).'

My brother left us way too soon. If I could capture even an ounce of the radiance his soul exuded, I will feel as though life has come full circle. Wherever you are, my love, my bhai, know that your Mashu misses you. I feel your presence, always.

Growing Up with My Dad

Karthika Satyanarayanan

Karthika is a biological sciences major from Krea University. She hopes to work in the field of infectious disease epidemiology some day. She is an ardent fan of the *Lord of the Rings* trilogy, black coffee and foosball.

Do you ever wonder what it's like to not have an ability you take for granted? I do, sometimes. That's because I live with someone who doesn't have something that I take for granted—the ability to use both legs properly. When my dad was little, he became really sick with polio. The sickness left him with a crippled left leg. Though my dad can walk, he can do so only with great difficulty. At home, my mom, my sister and I have always largely divided the house chores amongst us so my dad doesn't have to do anything that could strain his legs or tire him out. Now it's just my mom and my sister taking care of things, since I moved out a few months ago when I started college. I live in a hostel now. My mom is a student counsellor who used to be a lawyer. I'm mentioning the lawyer bit only because that's how she always introduces herself to people. My sister, who's in the eleventh grade, is the child every Indian parent hopes to have—she's smart, studious, and aspires to be a doctor. My sister and I do the laundry and the dishwashing, and my mom has always taken care of the cooking, grocery shopping and house repairs. When my dad can, he helps out with the laundry or dishwashing or by ordering groceries online when my mom cannot go out and do it. So, the daily functioning of our household is divided amongst us in a way where we have probably always taken a little bit more responsibility as children.

Whenever we go to Chennai to visit relatives—my grandparents and my parents' siblings and my cousins—they do whatever they can to make my dad feel as comfortable as possible, sometimes even overdoing with help that my dad feels he doesn't need. And this helpfulness doesn't stop with just the family. Whenever we travel, if my mom and sister and I are unable to help my dad up or down steep steps or slopes, strangers, who sometimes don't even speak the same language as us, are willing to carry my dad to help. Observing the ways in which people behave around my dad, it occurs to me that the idea of extending help to a person with a disability is differently motivated. My mom, my sister and I assist my dad with what he needs to complete a task, which otherwise he largely does on his own. I have noticed that other people sometimes undermine my dad's ability to function on his own and try to do everything for him, thinking that that is being helpful. The irony is that I used to think not so differently from these other people.

Actually, I don't remember thinking about my dad's disability when I was a kid; I'm not even sure I realised that my dad was disabled. But when I did, I assumed that that was what my dad's whole life was like. And somewhere in the back of my mind, I thought that my dad couldn't really do things for himself, because people always did everything for him. I thought that having a disability meant being completely dependent on the people around you and not being able to do anything for yourself. But I was mistaken.

When my dad was about five years old, his parents sent him from Chennai to live with his aunt in Delhi. They sent a little boy, who could not walk properly, who did not know how to speak English or Hindi, to live with people he'd never met before, because they were unable to handle my dad's disability—financially or emotionally. In Delhi, my dad did not get the help or attention he needed, because his aunt's family was a large one. They simply did not have the time to deal with him. So, basically, from the time my dad was five, till he got married, he managed most things on his own. He did really well in school—he spent all his free time poring over books since he couldn't go out and play like the other kids—and went on to study at the Indian Institute of Science, then he got his master's degree in the US, to become an engineer. It was after I learnt all of this that I realised the enormity of my incorrect assumption. I assumed that my dad was not an independent person without bothering to find out what his life is like from his point of view. I assumed that not being able to use both legs properly meant living a sad and deprived life without being able to do the things people with well-functioning legs can do. I felt like a horrible person for making such an assumption. Then I realised that I probably wasn't the only one to make such an assumption—not that that made me feel any better about myself. An essay I was required to read for one of my classes at college—'World into Word', by Mark Doty—got me thinking about it.* The essay is about the difficulties Doty faces as a writer trying to accurately experience and represent the world that he writes about. In one part of the essay, he writes about a visually impaired person called Stephen Kuusisto and an incident from his memoir, *Planet of the Blind*. Kuusisto talks about the

---

* This essay was originally the transcript of an audio assignment for my writing and oral communication class at college. I am so grateful to my professor, Dr Anannya Dasgupta, for helping me shape and edit the essay.

time he and his guide dog are lost in New York City's Grand
Central Station. Though Kuusisto describes the incident as an
exhilarating adventure, Doty is inclined to describe Kuusisto's
visual experience using words like 'only' and 'merely'. Like
me, Doty made assumptions about a person with a disability.
As a person with perfect sight, Doty assumed that the sight
of a visually impaired person is somewhat limited compared
to the sight of a visually unimpaired person, before trying to
understand what the world really looks like from Kuusisto's
point of view. He did change his views, though, once he
figured out that he was wrong.

I now realise that having a disability definitely does not
mean that the person is completely dependent on the people
around them. I'm not saying they're completely independent.
They do need help sometimes, like how my dad needs to hold
someone's hand to climb up or down the stairs when there
are no railings. But when you think about it, is anyone really
completely independent? We all need help for something or
another. It could be tying shoelaces, opening jars or even
financially. It's just that the needs of people with disabilities
are different from the needs of people without disabilities.
These needs are what set people with disabilities apart in the
eyes of people without disabilities. These needs are things
people without disabilities would never even register in their
minds as needs. This occurred to me while reading a letter
my dad had written to my mom when they were living in
different countries just after their engagement. I noticed that
my dad had spent several sentences marvelling at his luck
regarding the university he was attending for his master's
degree. The university he had got into had a flat campus,
while the one he was rejected from was in a hilly area. My
dad wrote how he would've found it extremely difficult to

walk around if he'd got into and attended the university with the hilly campus, and was so glad that he went to the other one. Flat campus versus hilly campus—that's a factor I would never have considered or even noticed, but for my dad, the terrain of the university campus affected his living.

Here's another question. What really is disability? I'm not sure. It's clearly not as simple as being unable to do something, because the world is built for people who can do the things that people with disabilities cannot do. The world we live in normalises the things associated with a majority of people and frowns upon, is confused by, and forms stereotypes of anything associated to a minority. People with disabilities are a minority and hence are treated with caution, as if they're fragile beings. When strangers offer to help my dad, their faces are full of pity. As someone who has lived with a person with a disability her whole life, I am certain when I say people with disabilities are not fragile or delicate—they just need some help to navigate a world that is not made for them. People without disabilities view people with disabilities as just disabilities; they fail to see the person in front. My dad's crippled leg doesn't make him any less of a dad. He is not defined by his disability. He is kind and intelligent and loves his kids and would do anything for them. He's someone who's worked hard to get where he is today. He's a bibliophile and a big fan of *Star Wars*. I hope I grow up to be like him.

People like me, who took their abilities for granted, but have also had the opportunity to care for and grow up with a person with a disability, have had the experience of learning empathy right at home. By which, I mean that I have had to understand my dad's world from his point of view. The most important thing that I have understood is that help that comes from a place of sympathy is about the person extending the help and how good they feel about it, whereas help that comes from a place of empathy is about the person who needs the help. It is the latter that keeps intact the dignity and the independence of the person with a disability.

Rock, Paper, Scissors

Shobhana Kumar

Shobhana Kumar's book of haibun, *A Sky Full of Bucket Lists*, is the recipient of the Honourable Mention in the Touchstone Distinguished Books Award, 2021. She has two collections of poetry and seven books covering memoirs, biographies and industrial histories. She works in the spaces of social work, education and branding.

There is a place somewhere between the gut and the diaphragm where the uneasiness begins. It is a slow, spiralling feeling that slaloms to the chest bone and locks itself right next to the heart. It is like a small boulder trapped in a crevice that pierces a vacant spot every time she inhales. It is the pain that keeps Kathyayini awake, lulls her to sleep and awakens her with a start. Thoughts run amok inside her. Every loved one's life ends dismally. Her own life is a static image of her waiting at the edge of a cliff, holding on to dear life against an unrelenting wind.

She surveys the room. The bed is positioned in the centre. Right above her is a thirty-five-year-old fan that whirrs incessantly, true to its long years of service, creaking occasionally but not once stopping. The sunlight glints through the thick pink cotton curtains, lending an almost-always sunset glow to the room. A harsh tube light blinks to life faithfully at 5.30 every evening, regardless of the season. An intravenous fluid stand is set beside the bed. The side table has three plastic boxes with medicines of every kind. Two large teakwood cupboards impose their presence in the far corner. An intricately carved dresser with a mirror and table completes the picture. This is a room that has seen better times.

The left side of her body feels numb and carries all the weight of her eighty-nine years. The gold, silks, world travel, VIP gatherings, ceremonies, tussles, wars with the in-laws, fights with the husband, four childbirths and two miscarriages have come to this. One perfectly working arm and leg. One dead. She mumbles as the left part of her lips stretches in unintelligible syllables. There's panic in the eyes and the hand seems to grasp at nothingness. The moan turns furtive, urgent. She manages to find the alarm button and repeatedly presses it.

Shanthi is in the kitchen, making the last batch of rasam podi for an order. The counter is a mess of concoctions and sweetmeats in various stages of preparation. The room is a contrast to the rest of the well-appointed house. It has not really been designed for modern living. On the large shelves and alcoves are haphazardly stacked vessels of every size. At one time, this kitchen had played host to all the weddings in the family. Food from here had always been a gift. Now, it works for her upkeep. Shanthi looks around and forces the past away from memory. She allows her mind to wander to her favourite place instead. She is in magical USA where, they say, machines do most of the work. She can smell it in the way the packaged almonds arrive. And, occasionally, some trivia for her. She may never know of life there, but decides that it is where she is going to be born the next time. The alarm drags her back to the heady aroma of spice.

It has been a long day. She sighs and moves toward the bedroom. A gush of antiseptic and phenyl-swept floors invades her olfactory senses. She inhales sharply as she bends down, looking at the anger in the eyes that meet hers. The hand on the bed yanks her hand to the open empty palm. The sounds from the throat are now guttural, primeval. It takes Shanthi a moment to understand what Kathyayini wants.

'It's right here,' she says. She reaches under the pillow and brings out a silk pouch and thrusts it into the impatient hand. 'Where will it go? Who is going to come and take it from you? Let me keep it in your cupboard at least.' Her tone is controlled anger, the kind that only the speaker knows of.

The hand is too busy fumbling through the silk. It feels the round, perfectly chiselled shape of the diamond ear stud. It feels another. And there's the three-stone-studded nose ring. Kathyayini is still angry that the pouch was not in her hands. Shanthi can make out this much.

'The doctor was here. You were sleeping. I did not want it to go missing.' Shanthi says, a wave of resentment welling up inside her. All these years of caring and this is what she gets. She leaves the still-mumbling Kathyayini and hastens to the kitchen. The tears have emptied themselves so much that all that remains is a dry pool of complete apathy. There are just chores. Chores of filial piety and chores of livelihood. Once you compartmentalise those, you just get on with it. Put emotion in between and never let it slice through either side. On the rare moments you have, you indulge in the happiness of wandering thought. But you always know that it must come down to these twin to-dos. There is no place for the future in this milieu. If the future is anything like the woman on the bed, Shanthi will gladly forgo it. Tomorrow is the 'now' in perennial loop.

Curious thing this sense of responsibility is. She was the least capable of her siblings, the least stable financially and yet, here she is, doing the work of care because there is no one else to do it. It is as simple as that. When there are too many takers for the picking, the last person has no choice, have they? There is only that, the last there is, to contend with. It is a while before she realises she is cursing under her breath. She likes to. It helps keep her sane.

The ceiling fan slowly whirs above Kathyayini's immobile limbs. It has been slowed as the temperature outside has dipped. She looks up, watching the shadows its blades cast upon the ceiling. She has stared into that vacant space for three years now. She remembers in the immediate aftermath of the fall, she had asked to turn the idiot box on at 7 a.m. every morning. The bespectacled man would have better prognosis for her star today. All the planets would be better aligned. She would get better. She would be able to go shopping again. After nine months, she knew the truth. The forecasts were a bunch of hogwash. All that had happened was the change of jewellery the astrologer wore. He seemed more animated than before and more convincing. But she was done believing. The stars had come full circle and decided to stay put at the worst alignment possible. She had then shifted her attention to mythological serials. But the gods had nothing to offer her. All their moralising was for mortals. They seemed to be able to get out of any trouble by the snap of their hands. She had cursed them out of her life too. The soaps had been more interesting. All the in-laws, busy plotting against each other. After two years, that faded too. Now, all she does is stare at the ceiling, repeatedly call out to hapless Shanthi, demand her favourite dishes and sleep. Through it all is one thought. If she lets go of all her life's savings, she will be thrown out in a minute. All the children are like that. And the daughters-in-law and sons-in-law are worse. She can't afford to let go. It is hers. Her body might have failed her but no one can do her out of all that she has so diligently put away.

Shanthi is almost done. All she needs to do is to pack the podi into the plastic covers and take it to the neighbouring grocers. He will run his fancy automatic machine on the edges and ensure the plastic congeals into a tight seal. But that will have to wait until tomorrow. Right now, there is just no energy. She turns on the gas stove and puts in two handfuls of oats into a pan of water. She absently stirs it, indulging the thought of how effective cyanide might be if mixed into it. She remembers the news article about the lady in Kerala who got away with seven murders. And here, no one would really know. There is no one to care enough. She smiles at such wickedness. In her head, she lists all the people she would give this imaginary mix of oats and cyanide. Her husband. Of course. First thing. The neighbour, who always wants her podis but never once offers to give her anything in return? Yes. Definitely. All the in-laws. Some of her own family members. Gosh, she would beat the Kerala lady, she thinks. She quickly chides herself, shuddering at how easily the mind can turn to villainy.

The oats taste like mud. Kathyayini plucks the plastic bowl from Shanthi's hands and flings it back at her, spitting out what still remains in her mouth. This is the tongue that has feasted on Thanjavur's famed delicacies. This is the tongue that has taught the hands to perfect how to make a paruppu payasam right, cook a five-course meal and still have the hands smelling of spices after a bath with Cinthol soap. This is the tongue that could tell the difference between fresh filter coffee and a day-old decoction. This is the tongue that had reduced the brides of the family to shuddering messes at the thought of serving her a meal. The blandness of the oats couldn't compare with the tastes she has feasted on. The oats deserve to be spat out.

White flecks splatter on Shanthi's greys, her face, the purple saree, her sweat-stained blouse and neck. It is all over the bed. She takes out a wet-wipe from the side table and begins mopping up the mess. She goes to the bathroom and cups her hands with water from the wash basin. She lets the water wash over her face and comes back. She says nothing. This has gone on for too long to react. There will be time for tears later. Some day, all this will be over.

Kathyayini has drifted off to sleep. In another world, the anklets on her toes tinkle as she walks. The two thick bands of toe-rings clink in symphony with the anklets. The maroon sheen of her Kanjeevaram rustles against her brisk step. And then she accidentally trips over a pot of water. Her eyelids flutter open. Her nostrils gag at the overpowering smell of ammonia. The bed around her hips is moist and fluid seeps from the rubber sheet on to the mattress. The tears come pouring down. She raises her hand and slaps her forehead repeatedly. The wailing is that of a death house. Her hands tremble as she reaches for the alarm bell. They wade through the waste, find it and press it.

Shanthi rushes to the bedside and throws open the sheet. She shushes her in urgent tones and calms her down. She turns her to the left, all the time trying to pull the soiled bed sheet out from underneath her. The woman on the bed weighs a tonne; she only looks frail. Shanthi peels off the diaper and grabs a bunch of wet-wipes to clean her up. The entire task takes twenty minutes, maybe more than that, but who's looking. She takes the bed sheet and dunks it in a bucket of water. She makes a mental note to ask for more diapers to be sent by the visiting son next month. The local ones are no good. They always manage to leak. She empties a couple of capfuls of Dettol in the bucket and lets the sheets soak. As she rinses them, the alarm bell goes off again.

Anything can happen. Kathyayini knows this. She can be strangled to death and no one will know. She can be snuffed out with a pillow pressed to her face. Or be simply left to die. There is nothing left. But Shanthi won't let her go like that.

Kathyayini has given her too much. For too long in her life. This is just payback time. It is going to be okay. She presses the button and calls out her name, muffled as it is, but over and over again until the familiar face stares back at her.

Shanthi brings back the silken pouch, smelling of Dettol, and transfers the contents to an old cotton potli (bag). She runs a safety pin to fasten it to the cotton nighty. She refuses to make eye contact. She empties the oats into the kitchen bin and comes back with a glass of Ensure. She spoons it into the invalid's mouth. This time, there is no fuss. No conversation.

Nine months later, it all comes to a grand finale. A quiet one, actually. Kathyayini slowly slips into a peaceful, eternal trance. The doctors say it is a miracle she has even lived this long. The eyes are donated. The other organs are too old for anyone else. At the funeral, everyone pats Shanthi and tells her they wish they had a daughter like her. Her brothers, it is clear, are getting increasingly bored with the slowness of things in India.

Shanthi packs some of her delicacies into three separate parcels—one for each of her brothers. They are flying back the next day. And then she pulls out the cotton potli from within the folds of her saree blouse. 'This is Amma's,' she says. 'Do what you want with it. I have no use for these things.'

The house is strangely empty and quiet after they are gone. Her husband is off to work as usual. Shanti pulls out the old steel trunk from under her cot and finds the family album. She spends two happy hours diligently cutting her mother out of every single picture.

BOOK SIX

Creating Roadmaps and Spaces

Note

The rate of burnout among special educators is higher than that found in most other professions. What is perhaps worse is that the world dresses them in the same invisibility cloak with which it dresses persons with disabilities and their families. A special educator typically works with a range of disabilities. To be effective, they have to customise their teaching to suit each student's learning style. As Nirmala Pandit says, it is important to observe the child carefully before arriving at teaching or intervention methods. It is also important to explain to the child what his or her learning style is. Navigating this complex terrain of offering learning support to young people with disabilities is often done without a map, as Poonam Natarajan points out. New roadmaps are created along the way.

Namita Jacob, founder of Chetana, argues that one of the lessons that special education teaches is that changing the life of even one person can make a difference and that often it is about asking yourself what is the one thing that needs to be adjusted in order for things to become accessible for a person with disability.

An individualised education programme is not easy to deliver. Inclusive classrooms that comprise both students with different learning styles and neurotypical students pose a different kind of challenge altogether. Here, the teacher will also have to sensitise the latter to classmates who learn and develop differently. The work of a special educator is very different from that of most other teachers. The latter may not quite see them as colleagues. Given that special educators typically work with smaller groups, focus on skills rather than content, and work with students who are perceived as 'slow', their work may be perceived as being easier or less important. As Lakshmi points out in her interview, they have to deal with the mainstream school system that literally casts out children with different learning styles, resulting in missed learning opportunities that take a lot of work to address, not to mention psychological scars. They may also have to deal with parents (and sometimes extended family members) who are either disinterested and uninvolved, in denial or in grief, or simply very overprotective of their child.

In the end, it is often the children themselves who prove to be the best guides. As Poonam Natarajan, founder of Vidya Sagar, says, it is children and their specific needs out of which they developed whole new programmes. She argues that a trans-disciplinary approach is important, as is the understanding that we learn from one another. Poonam also points out that special educators and therapists must ultimately work with parents and train them so that they can support their child, and that therapeutic interventions ought not be mystified. She argues that therapy will work only if it becomes a way of life, and therefore the parent needs to be equipped with the skills of a therapist or special educator.

Not surprisingly, many special educators and people who work in the broader field of disability services also happen to be family members. This tends, typically, to be mothers, as is the case with Geethanjali Rajan, Poonam Natarajan and Sumithra Prasad, but also, as is the case with Amaresh, the child of people with disabilities. All of them have experienced or perceived a gap in the sort of support their son, daughter or parent requires and so are drawn, almost naturally, to the field.

Sumithra Prasad, founder of Society All Inclusive bakery, has realised that one of the biggest challenges that a person with developmental disability faces is the lack of a network of friends. It is with this in mind that SAI bakery has put in place a buddy system.

Special educators are sometimes drawn to the field because they too have struggled with the school system. Nirmala Pandit says: 'When I was in school, people thought I was not a good enough student. I could never be taught. I had to learn on my own. I used to question the ones who came first in class, "How do you learn?" They used to say, "We don't read the whole chapter." I never knew how to game the system. There was a girl in my class who I used to write essays for every day. Later, I realised that she perhaps didn't know how to write at all! We all have learning issues! The borders are very thin.'

Much more so than others in the field of education, special educators have to be agile learners, open to a sort of continuous learning, to figuring things out as they go along, looking to the child to create learning programmes and altering the metrics used for assessments.

Breaking Wave

Geethanjali Rajan

Geethanjali Rajan has taught in schools, colleges and in an open-school environment in Chennai. She is trained to remediate Specific Learning Difficulties and is happiest in a class filled with diverse learning needs.

What is worse: you love words desperately but are unable to use them appropriately, or you love words desperately but are told that you don't know how to use them appropriately?

The answer to this question doesn't matter. Like dyslexia or dysgraphia or dyscalculia or dyspraxia, it is one of those conundrums without a 'correct' answer.

Coming from a family of educators, I didn't think twice about getting into training and teaching as a career. It didn't matter what I taught; I was quite sure that I wanted to teach. My meaningful engagement with teaching, however, started rather late, after my training in 'special education', where I learnt how to teach children with SLDs. The term is a convenient collective noun—mostly used to group together any individual learning style that a traditional system considers unproductive, at least in most of India. I personally dislike the last alphabet of SLD—the 'd' for disability. When a difference is severe enough that it disables, it is termed a disability, but when the term is used too early, too soon or too loosely, as it is used more often than not, it ends up disabling an individual.

My daughter survived many months of a traumatic intrauterine environment and when she was born, the family did a little dance because she was fully formed. It was nothing short of a miracle. When she started playschool, she was quite a linguist, reeling off, in enviably perfect pronunciation, English, Malayalam, Tamil and Japanese names of animals and numbers, charming everyone with her stories and questions. All well till there. Then started the system of formal education—the nightmare (for any three-year-old) of having to start writing the entire alphabet in capital and small letters. We lasted a mere three months in the system. That was all it took to destroy a fun-loving three-year-old and turn her into a fearful, timid and reticent being.

A quick shift to the Montessori system helped salvage her spirit. A very observant and sensitive environment led us to evaluations and assessments with specialists and a whole Pandora's box opened up. Very often, parents want a precise diagnosis about their child. So did I, but I never got a precise answer, only the word 'co-morbidity'. No one could point out what was wrong or how wrong. Those were dark days. I didn't know if she was physically unwell or mentally unwell or just not capable of academic work. Looking back, it didn't matter, but at that point, matter it did. Before the age of six, no one can tell if a child has dyslexia. One can only say that a child is 'at risk for SLD'. So there we were—'at risk'.

A very senior educator assessed my daughter, and her advice is what has seen us through all these years of formal education. She pointed us to what is called 'occupational therapy', which helps to strengthen muscles, gross motor movements, fine motor movements, balance and all the other skills that a human being needs before actually sitting down to write legibly on paper. This was the best thing that could happen to my daughter. The next ten years, we worked on her joints and muscles, her posture and balance—my daughter gained health and I learnt patience. We also forayed into *kalaripayattu*, a martial art which originated in Kerala and helped her body and her balance. Later, in her teen years, she moved to weight training, tai-chi and yoga, to help her deal with her physical development. Even with all this, she was at a height that just passed muster and a weight that had people think she was a good five years younger than her age. Now, out of her teens, she is considered tall (suddenly!). Thanks to all this, we gave our child the gift of better physical health.

The journey through the many systems, subjects and schools has led me to more learning than I could have had with a child that fit in well, was run of the mill and aced everything dished out to her. (I am quite confident that this kind of child does not exist, though many parents won't agree with me.) My angst and anger at the system slowly turned into strategies to deal with it. Here, I also believe that the 'system' is made by people and of people. The strategies which parents need are essentially those that will help the child cope with the system and its people, and not just cope with the academic difficulties. My experiences have been a mixed bag—from encouraging principals, kind teachers and learning-centre educators who firmly believe in children's abilities to insensitive individuals who publicly shame children, call them 'lazy' and role-model bully behaviour. I have been fortunate to see behaviour patterns that I would like to model and those that I would never want anyone to face, definitely not a child with dyslexia. As a parent, I have had to hone my interpersonal skills to a level beyond the professional, to deal with the myriads of people in my daughter's life—principals, teachers, doctors, therapists, other parents—just to ensure survival in the system.

Dealing with the education system—the board, the assessments and the tests were the easier part—we did

Montessori, the state board, CBSE and the National Institute of Open Schooling (NIOS). The last was an absolute blessing because studying subjects that interested her made my daughter do extremely well academically, leading her to develop confidence and motivation. Here, I have been fortunate to find some un-winged angels in the form of remedial teachers, learning centre heads, therapists and doctors. They didn't underplay the condition, but neither did they overdo the labelling.

When I decided to train as a special educator (again, a term that I am not too fond of—shouldn't all educators in a system be 'special'?), I did so with the rather narrow scope of understanding what tools and skills I could use to help my daughter. But two days into the course and I knew it was what would take me onto the path of actually facilitating learning. What I had been doing till then was training young and not-so-young adults in language and soft skills. I would 'deliver' a package, a lesson or a concept to a captive audience with no hope of escape from the classroom. What I started doing from then on, was to actually reach out to the learner and help them engage with the content in a way that suited them and hence, helped them learn better. When I taught the NIOS syllabus in a mainstream school, I found that my students were my greatest teachers. Each had a different learning style, source of motivation and sense of achievement. One instance that will never leave me was a celebration of my birthday. My class of fourteen-year-olds arranged a surprise party for me with cake, flowers, portraits drawn by the more artistic ones, and music. Needless to say, it was against the rules but we were all forgiven when the head teacher found out that the class of 'different learners' had executed a brilliant event management project all by themselves! What better proof that the home science teacher had succeeded in teaching them that part of the syllabus well!

In all these years, the greatest lessons have been to work with the learner's strengths. In my case, my daughter is highly drawn to colours and she paints as well. This became a medium to express herself as well as a tool for learning, where she would make her own diagrams to learn concepts. If a child has to learn a concept, repeating it (in an increasingly higher volume) is not going to be as helpful as letting them learn it through their own strengths. Of course, it takes time, effort and a lot of luck to find out what works for each child. But that is the game of SLD—a waiting game, a patience game, a game of slowing down the pace of learning if needed and not necessarily speeding up the child. My discussions with parents and stakeholders in the education system often revolve around changing their expectations from the child. After all, we are the adults in the environment—shouldn't we be the ones to adapt to the child, rather than expecting the child to adapt to a hardened system?

The biggest challenge for me has been one of social acceptance of a child with differences. When parents slowly learn that the child is not the same thing as her academic achievement, they start to accept the child. However, SLD has a very great social challenge component, where the child's self-esteem is often sacrificed at the altar of coping with academics. This, in turn, leads to challenges in socialising with peers. It doesn't help that, typically, peers aren't sensitised to differences—this being a bane of our times. Very often, I have had to step in to resolve bullying and name-calling. What makes us raise children to believe that they are superior because they do not need academic support? The very same 'ordinary' children go to tuition centres or coaching centres for academic support to get into a college. That is considered superior but academic support at an earlier age is not. These are common issues that parents of children with SLD face—I am no different.

Today, my daughter hopes to champion the cause of dyslexia (we still don't know if she has dyslexia, dyspraxia or dysgraphia ... but for convenience, we call it dyslexia) and a theme I constantly hear from her is that kids should be allowed to be different. We still don't know if the labelling has helped or harmed her. The jury is out on that, especially since in college more than half the class has issues related to language acquisition, expression and, of course, math. Perhaps the world has many more children with dyslexia than we know—a fortunate thing, if they are all as sensitive and creative as many of the kids I have seen! Meanwhile, my daughter also says that there is far too much stigma around the label; many who hear from her that she has a difficulty treat her like she is terminally ill, while others tell her that it will go away soon. Wrong, on both counts. We have also had many humorous conversations around whether she should 'come out of the closet'. Jokes apart, most kids do not want to be identified as having a learning difficulty. They just want to be the same as every other kid. Very few will stand up and say that they have a difficulty—my daughter has reached a point of 'if you don't have dyslexia, don't comment'.

The emotions that have been mine the last twenty years are similar to the ones that any other parent might have had. There have been times when I have had to stand by my child and fight the world and there have been times of endless laughter and infinite joy. But if I were to attribute all of this to the diagnosis of SLD, that would be a very narrow world view indeed. Whether your child is a high achiever in academics or sports, a child who doesn't know what they are good at, a child with a diagnosis of diabetes or an adopted child, we all ride the same rollercoaster. Fortunately, I am a writer also and many of those emotions find their way into my writing. However, the genre that I write—haiku—is not one that encourages an outpouring of emotion, and I am thankful for that too!

Dyslexia is a very subjective and individualistic condition, not a generic disease that requires standard treatment. That I have had to treat my child in a way that is different from the way a neighbour would treat their child, is probably the better way to parent—tailor the means to the child.

If I had to choose an easier life for myself, I would. There is nothing to be got from pointless struggles against a system. But if I had to choose between teaching children in a plain old class and teaching children with SLD, I would choose the latter—they are fun, bright, interesting, different and, speaking very selfishly, they have kept me young and smiling. As a parent, if I had to choose between a child with SLD and one without, I would choose one who is as fun, witty, interesting, different, quirky and sensitive as my daughter—SLD or not. It doesn't matter.

A Language in Its Own Right

An Interview with
Amaresh Gopalakrishnan

Amaresh Gopalakrishnan has over twenty years of experience in the field of special education, sign language research, and training and sign language interpreting.

Srilata: As I understand it, your parents are both hearing impaired. Is that what brought you to the field of special education and sign language research and interpretation?

Amaresh: Being a CODA, that is, a Child of Deaf Adults, I have been brought up in the deaf world right from birth. My parents made sure that I was not taken away by my hearing (non-deaf) grandparents or relatives, as was usually the case with other deaf parents. In this way, I was completely immersed in their world and had the benefit of learning sign language from birth. As I grew up, I was exposed to other spoken languages through my neighbourhood peers and school. So, I was multilingual from a very early age.

My father is the founder-member of the Madras Association of the Deaf and even before that, he was involved with other associations for the deaf for a long time. Thus, I was taken to all events and meetings for the deaf from a very early age. I would also interpret for my parents and other deaf friends of theirs. In this sense, you could say that I have been in this field since birth. As I grew up to be a teenager, I got more interested in other things, and my role was taken up by my younger sister. However, when I was in Coimbatore for an internship in 1998, my father was invited to a conference hosted by the Sri Ramakrishna Mission Vidyalaya College of Education. It was a three-day affair, and on the request of my father, I attended the conference on the third day. They needed an interpreter during the seminar, and as I knew how to sign, I was asked to step in. This was the first time I formally interpreted at a conference. At the end of the event, the principal of the college received positive feedback from participants about my interpreting skills, and he immediately offered me a job as a project assistant to create the first Indian sign language dictionary. I took a while to accept his offer as I had been planning a career in the field of computer science, but in November 1998, I joined the project. It could be said this was my launchpad in the field of hearing impairment.

Srilata: What was it like growing up as the hearing child of deaf parents? Did you feel like you had a certain responsibility towards your parents? Was there sometimes a kind of reversal of roles?

Amaresh: In my early days, I did not distinguish that I had deaf parents, while others had hearing parents. Whenever I was with my parents, I used to sign and with others, I used voice. Only much later in my childhood did I realise that I was a different child, probably because I was treated differently in school. Whenever I got into trouble at school, I was not punished as much as the other students were. And I also learnt that my sister and I got a concession in the school fees due to our parents' disability. That was probably the time I felt that I was a bit different from other students, and also 'special', in a sense. Not much later, I felt I had some additional responsibilities other than just studying and playing when I realised that I had to act as a translator for my parents. I used to go to the shop a lot to buy provisions;

I had to act as the communicator when we got our very first telephone at home, during visits to our family doctor, at school meetings, when we had visitors at home or when there was a salesman at our door, and with the neighbours. Introverted by nature, I did not like doing all those things, and I would invariably ask my younger sister to do them. It was when I became involved in the field that I realised I had a much bigger responsibility—not only towards my parents but also towards the whole deaf community. My father has been very much involved in welfare activities for the deaf from an early age, and this example influenced me a lot to bring about positive change in every way I could.

Srilata: There are two schools of thought regarding language for the hearing impaired—the speech therapy approach trains them to 'speak' like hearing people, while the sign language approach involves a whole other language. What is your take on these approaches?

Amaresh: The oral-aural method is just a communication modality, while sign language is a complete language in itself. Speech therapy can be given to anyone who has problems with speech, not just the deaf. Learning how to speak is an added skill that the deaf can achieve through speech therapy. Auditory training needs to be given to those hearing-impaired people who have some residual hearing and can hear sounds using a hearing aid or with a cochlear implantation. And this needs to be done at a very early age. This too, in a way, is an added skill.

On the other hand, sign language is a language that each and every deaf person must learn to be able to develop other sets of skills, like learning spoken language, reading and writing spoken language, and receiving speech and auditory training. In my view, forcing deaf children to speak by giving speech therapy without the foundation of sign language should be considered a violent act, as the child has absolutely no idea what he is being forced to do. In this case, the deaf child often suffers mentally—and physically as well. I have heard stories of deaf children having their hands bound in an effort to force them to use speech. They aren't given any choice; in this sense, it could be perceived as a violent act. However, if the child has a foundation of sign language and the speech therapist is able to communicate with the child in sign language, it creates a comfortable environment for the child as s/he understands what is required of him/her. In this way, you aren't forcing the child, but helping the child to develop their speech skills. A language is vital for overall development, wherein to be able to speak is an added advantage. This is my take.

Srilata: What are some of the most important things people outside the deaf community need to know about sign language in general? How does it handle complex concepts, abstract ideas, regional differences in language, slang, pitch and tone?

Amaresh: The most important thing people need to understand is that sign language is a language in its own right. Though it is a visual language and uses the hands, body, face and space, it has all the elements of a spoken language, including grammar. One can express oneself in sign language just as much as in spoken languages. Since sign language is a proper language, as with other languages, it also has its own regional dialects and variations. However, this does not hinder deaf people from forming strong communities, and in this age of technological advancements, which have made communication much easier for deaf people, deaf communities from different parts of India are able to easily converse with each other. The complexities, if any, are yet to be analysed and documented. Pitch and tone in sign language are indicated by facial expressions, body movements and the speed of movement of the hands.

Every Child Has a Background Story

A Conversation with
Lakshmi Krishnakumar

Lakshmi Krishnakumar is the director at Sankalp, an open school based in Chennai that caters to children with learning disabilities.

Srilata: Tell me a little about Sankalp and the work you do.

Lakshmi: The first thing to keep in mind when it comes to SLD or dyslexia is that there are no quick solutions. It is an inherent difficulty that is often compounded by the child's environment. We have to understand which is the bigger problem. Only when we start working with the child do we come to know if the problem is created, if it is an external one. If you find yourself not making any progress with the child, if the gap between what she should be able to do and what she is actually doing begins to widen, that is the time to come up with another plan of action.

We are trained to handle SLD, dyslexia and other processing disorders. But the majority of the children who come to us suffer from environment-related problems, lack of exposure or cognitive challenges that may be more severe—when you talk about SLD or dyslexia, you know that the child has average or more than average intelligence.

We have to be tuned to understand the child. Sometimes, training and textbook knowledge are not enough. We may know a lot of theory but we need to adapt to the situation. The strength of our classrooms are not more than ten children. Even then, the differences between the children are really wide. There's no one size fits all.

Srilata: If we were to think of it as multiple intelligences, would that work better? If we were to place children in environments where their particular kind of intelligence is able to blossom, wouldn't that be good?

Lakshmi: I do agree. But is there any change happening in our educational system? Not really! There's this huge gap between what the child can do and what is expected of him or her. Why don't we use other parameters and measures to assess children? Why don't we assess them on the basis of their dance, music or cooking—if that is where their interest lies? If they learn the vocabulary that forms part of a play, why can't we assess them on that? Nothing like that is happening. So, the theory of multiple intelligences really works but do our curricula and evaluations cater to that? We hear pathetic stories of schools just sending some children out because their pass percentage has come down. Schools don't like children who perform poorly. They don't tell the parents this directly, which is even sadder. They inform us and place the responsibility on us to tell the parents. They say, 'We can't keep this child any longer. You please take care of him or her,' and they send the child to us. The parents then approach us with an assessment—the IQ or aptitude report. This is typically done outside of school. The parents have not been told what the child's strengths are and so on. Why can't society become more sensitive? A lot of children who come to us have gone through so much trauma. Their parents have no say in this and are helpless. It is hard for them even to open up and say, 'I want the best for my child. This system is not working, so what's next?' The system pushes the children till class eight or nine, and after that no one knows what to do with them. Some children who come to us at this point can't even identify alphabets! The gap is so huge that we are not able to make up for it. Then we have to tell the parents there is only this much we can do. They don't understand when we tell them this.

Srilata: At what age are children typically referred to you?

Lakshmi: These days we have younger children of around eight or nine coming to us. This is far easier for us. But they already come, mind you, with a gap of four or five years, because they have not been exposed to a play school prior to this. Their basic skills are not developed. They suffer from this lack of exposure.

Srilata: What's the best window of opportunity for children with SLD?

Lakshmi: Eight or nine years should be okay. But I would go even further and recommend that they be assessed and identified when they are in kindergarten. This is never done.

Srilata: Tell me about your work with the children of Sankalp. Are there any incidents that stand out in your memory?

Lakshmi: We have this very intelligent child. Somewhere in his early years, he developed some fears. He was hyperactive. The parents took him to a psychiatrist who started medicating him heavily. He received a huge list of about ten medicines! He came to us much later, when he was about ten or eleven. Prior to that, he had been on this cocktail of medicines. Now this child gets quite aggressive. If he doesn't get his way, he flies into a rage and throws things around, but I can't blame him because his behaviour is triggered by the medication. He comprehends and reads well. His writing is not okay because of these medications. He has some motor difficulties and can't stand properly. He also has a lot of behavioural issues.

One day, some of our teachers came to me and said, 'How can we keep him here?' The boy had thrown something at one of our teachers. She had had a narrow escape and needed stitches. The teachers' point was that this was a safety issue, that other parents would talk about it and so on. 'What about the safety of other children?' they asked. But I stuck to my guns. I said, 'Let us not talk about this child. Let us sensitise the other children. They too have to understand him. These are things we can never teach them through textbooks. Experience is a better teacher. Even if we send him out, tomorrow there may be another child with similar issues.' Values are taught only through experience—not through a moral science class. I asked the teachers, 'What have you learnt from the incident? What are we going to teach the children? We have to teach them to look at life from another person's perspective. Look at the agony of the parents. They are under severe stress. They came to us with such trepidation.' So, we ended up keeping the child on. We gave him two breaks. The first time around, we referred him out for some physical training and then took him back. There was another episode involving this child. At that time, his parents had stopped taking him for physical training.

We offer this child a lot of flexibility. We allow him to come late. At Sankalp, he tries to be alert (he is drowsy because of the medications), tries to make friends.

Srilata: So, you are dealing with a spectrum of issues.

Lakshmi: Yes, a spectrum. We deal with all sorts of co-morbidities. It is difficult, sometimes, to understand what is at the root of a problem ... Another child came to us when he was very young. He had speech problems but was very intelligent. His father was very understanding but the mother had issues herself. She couldn't accept the fact that her son was like this. She went through some depression. She claimed

Sankalp was not doing anything for the child and said she was tired of us calling her in for discussions. So, I said, fine, if you are not happy, you can take the child out.

She pulled him out of Sankalp and the child went from the frying pan to the fire. When the father contacted me again, I told him that he should take his wife for psychiatric help. She was getting a bit violent with the child. They did all that and were very happy with the progress. The doctor asked them to send the child back to us. But he had lost so much ground by then! I discovered during my conversations with his father that the child's maternal grandmother was a very dominating person. The father told me that his wife went entirely by what her mother said. So now I am trying to get the grandmother into the picture. I have asked the father to bring her to meet us. This child is already thirteen and he is only ready for grade five. Ideally, he should be in the seventh or eighth grade. The fifth grade is the lowest grade we can keep him in. If he is placed in a class lower than this, it will affect his self-esteem. All his classmates have moved on.

Every child has got a background story. There are so many people involved. At the end of the day, there is nothing drastic you can do to change things. But you can at least give them hope. Some cases just seem so hopeless. There is no way the child is going to clear the tenth or the twelfth, which is what the parents are dreaming of. But we all live on hope, don't we?

Srilata: How and when did you enter this field?

Lakshmi: My background is in psychology. Entering this field just happened. I didn't plan it. It was clear though that I would not work with very severe challenges. I started work in 1991. I didn't know that there was something called learning disability. At the time, the discipline didn't say much about this area. I found it fascinating and was able to identify with some of the challenges that were described. I found myself wishing that I had been aware of this earlier—I would have been a more confident person! When I started doing psychological assessments, I began to observe scattered scores and had to come to conclusions on that basis. It was an organic process. I trained on the job.

I am currently interested in the idea of developmentally appropriate experiences. Young children, for instance, should be allowed to spill food so they can then figure out what to do. Instead of that, we hand them a napkin!

A Hidden Disability Is Very Difficult to Understand

A Conversation with Nirmala Pandit

Nirmala Pandit is a senior special educator who has worked with children with SLD. She is one of the founder-members of the Madras Dyslexia Association.

Srilata: Tell me about yourself. When and how did you enter the field of special education? What was the field like at the time? How has it changed since? Tell me about the Madras Dyslexia Association (MDA), which you founded.

Nirmala: I am one of those lucky people who have found a vocation that is more a passion than a job. I have always been very interested in how a person learns academically as well as experientially. I have also been very fond of children, looking for chances to babysit even as a young girl. I knew I wanted to teach, but not in a regular classroom. When I got a chance, I went to the USA to do special education, where I specialised in teaching children with hearing impairments and learning disabilities. This was in the early 1970s, when learning disabilities was a comparatively new field in the USA. On my return to India, I worked in a special school and then started my own practice.

My private practice dealt largely with children in mainstream schools who were finding academic learning difficult. In those days, there was hardly any awareness of SLDs. If a child did not cope well in school, he was deemed a slow learner or lazy. The idea that a child who was verbal and seemed intelligent and physically fit could still have a specific difficulty in academics was beyond most people's understanding. So, such children did not receive the help and encouragement that they deserved. These children fell between the cracks and suffered socially and, worse still, emotionally. It was an uphill task to convince parents, grandparents and schools that they needed to use a different approach to teach and nurture such children. Only with a lot of counselling and actual demonstration of how a child with an SLD learns and should be taught could they be convinced.

The scenario has changed considerably over the years, with more special educators and other such professionals entering the field, and with lobbying in the states and the Centre for recognition and the granting of examination provisions and a choice of subjects in the various boards. SLDs have finally been recognised and have found a place in the Rights of Persons with Disabilities Act of 2016. Of course, we have a long way to go. We need to be ever-evolving in our methods and, most importantly, vigilant that our children receive what has been promised.

I remember being asked by a senior education authority that he wanted to meet a child with SLD so that he could understand what such children look like! This was in the 1990s. A hidden disability is very difficult to understand.

Srilata: Did you work with a variety of learning disabilities or was your work confined largely to dyslexia?

Nirmala: I learnt about hearing impairments and SLD in training. I met a child with autism for the first time in my life when one was brought to our university clinic as a potential case of hearing impairment; this led me to do research and learn more about autism. Over the course of my career, I have taught academics to children with autism who were enrolled in mainstream schools.

Srilata: How would you explain dyslexia to a layperson? Have you ever felt the inadequacy of a word like 'dyslexia', felt that just one word is not enough to describe all the sorts of things that are going on in a person's life, especially when it comes down to how they learn? Do you think that the diagnosis of dyslexia can sometimes cut both ways? As in, it has its obvious advantages but the labelling can carry with it a certain sort of stigma too?

Nirmala: This is a very important question. There is a constant debate in our field about 'labelling' a child. I will explain my point of view. When parents want a consultation with me, I first request both of them and any other caretaker to meet me without the child present. This is a crucial meeting that involves the building up of trust and ensuring of confidentiality. I arrange the seats in a circle; there is no table between them and me—we are in this together. There is specific information to be gathered for me to understand them and the child, but it is gathered conversationally, not as a question-and-answer session. The parents are free to talk as much as they want to, no judgements are made, no opinions given. If I get the impression that the child needs an assessment, I explain why I feel so. I also explain the kind of assessment I will conduct, and counsel them on how to prepare the child for the session. I specifically assure the parents of children with SLD that in case their child needs help, help will be given and together we will see to it that the child becomes a confident learner and a happy person.

In case I feel that another professional should also be consulted, like a speech therapist or an occupational therapist, I refer them to one I have confidence in and provide them with an introductory and explanatory letter. I also make a call to the person later. After the assessment, if the child is found to have SLD, the condition is explained to the parents. Since SLD consists of multifarious facets and no two people are affected in the same way, it is important to first explain what the findings are. For example, is it the reading (dyslexia), the writing (dysgraphia) or maths (dyscalculia) that is difficult? Explanation has to be given as to which aspect of reading, writing or math is affected and which aspects are the strengths of the child. Then the underlying neurological aspect should be explained in simple terms: is it visual or auditory perception and processing or both that is the cause? How does the child learn, what is his or her learning style and how can we use it? Importantly, I emphasise that this is not an intellectual disability but a learning disability. The emotional and social aspects are also discussed. When the condition is explained with reference to the child and by drawing examples from what the parents have already observed, it is easier for us to explain and for them to understand.

It is very important to involve parents in the explanation. This has helped with all the parents I have counselled, whatever their background. I particularly discuss the strengths the child has—academically, socially, physically or emotionally. His talents, likes and dislikes are also discussed. When the condition is given a name, I find that parents as well as older children and adults are relieved. This is because they are assured that it is common and that they are not the only ones to face this difficulty. They also feel that a cause has been found and now work can be done to alleviate it. So, a 'label' helps. I also counsel the parents on how to help the child with academics, executive functions such as time management and prioritising and any other aspects that may go with the difficulty. I strongly feel that parents should be helped so that they can advocate for their child. They should be able to explain their child's strengths and needs to the school especially.

I make it a point to tell parents that I will be using the term SLD in the report and why it is necessary. In today's scenario, cumulative reports are required for a child to seek exam provisions in the board exams. Therefore, the term has to necessarily appear in the reports.

There is another issue too which needs attention. SLD has been erroneously categorised under intellectual disabilities, which is something we are contesting. It is actually a separate category.

Unless people start looking at differences without prejudice, things won't change to the extent we would like them to. We have to try and educate people that being different is okay. Any one of us could become disabled. In my old age, I realise how many disabilities we have. I wear a hearing aid and can't type for long. We should not look down upon someone who is young and can't do the same things, then. There should be no prejudice or stigma. It can happen to any one of us. People with disabilities should be accepted fully.

What we are doing solidly are awareness programmes in workplaces, in schools, etc., so what we find is that mostly in schools the ideas are coming up. They have resource rooms and also the CBSE has made a rule that all schools should have a special educator and counsellor. The problem is that all of this is available mostly only on paper. So, we have to be very vigilant that these provisions are given. Where do we see ramps, for instance? Now and then we see things like news in sign language, but it is not a regular feature. Whenever I look at coins, I always wonder how a visually impaired person is able to figure out the denominations. So, everything is difficult in day-to-day life. Especially now, very few people are working with disabilities in the workplace. So, I sometimes work with high functioning autistic children and try to place them in jobs. At one point, we were trying to place a non-verbal child. We could tell that he had the intellectual capacity. So, we put him through NIOS, though everybody said what is the point putting him through this. He got permission to take his exams on the computer. But in those days they were not allowed to use the computer so we went to The Spastics Society of TamilNadu (SPASTN) and they were kind enough to put us in touch with the director and we got permission for that child to use the computer. But a person had to sit by him and transcribe everything he had written on the computer onto paper! But recently, I heard that they can just turn in their computer exam. So, it is changing, but in bits and pieces. No one is looking at it holistically. Now we are trying to figure out what we can do. Where to get him trained? Whenever we approach people who say they will train him, it is the usual thing, like basket weaving—nothing intelligent, where the child uses his mind. So yes, there's a lot left to do. And then there is the social aspect. We may manage to place people with disabilities in a job but unless everyone in that particular workplace or institution are given vigorous training, it won't work.

Srilata: What tools do you use to assess a child who is brought in to meet you? Is there such a thing as the *degree* to which a child has dyslexia? How is that understood?

Nirmala: Unfortunately, we do not have satisfactory assessment tools that have been standardised on Indian children. There are a couple but they do not cover all the aspects. So, we mostly use tools from other countries such as the USA. We are careful in using these to make sure that we circumvent cultural biases, such as concepts or terms which are very foreign to our children. English is a foreign language to most of the children, so we have to be extra careful to differentiate between a true learning difficulty and difficulties arising from English as a second language. Ideally, the child should also be tested in their local language or mother tongue. The MDA has developed a teaching tool in Tamil. An assessment tool is yet to be developed. But we are able to tell whether a child has a genuine difficulty with the tools we use, through a differential diagnosis approach.

The tests allow us to classify degrees of difficulty as mild, moderate and severe. Here again, there are several factors to be considered. During our assessments it is very important to observe very closely how the child works. The assessment should not be about arriving at scores; it should be a study of the strategies he uses, attention levels, frustration levels, learning style, the questions he asks, independence versus dependence and many such factors.

I also like to do some diagnostic teaching during the session, where I teach a small skill, such as syllabication in spelling or how to read a math problem, to study how he picks it up and if it is based on his learning style. Then I explain to him what his style of learning is. The child gains confidence that he can indeed learn if shown how, and will use the strategy in the future. Thus, we find the degree of difficulty and how the child is dealing with it. The study of the personality of the child is very important as it tells us how he will help himself if shown how.

Srilata: Are you always able to tell what sorts of strategies will help the child you are working with? Tell me about some unusual strategies you have come up with.

Nirmala: The teaching strategies are decided both by the child's personal learning style as well as what must necessarily be taught within a certain skill. Both have to be kept in mind. The child must be taught to discipline his mind. The whole intent of remedial teaching is to develop an independent learner who understands that there are several strategies that can be used and how and when to use a particular strategy. Our interaction with the child in our care is personal and full of mutual respect. Since we work so closely with an individual, it is easy to understand him better.

One strategy that comes easily to mind is from several years ago, when I taught a child in class five. He used to struggle with the spelling of the English language as well as Hindi, which is a highly phonetic language. His favourite subject was history. I decided to abandon phonetic spelling for a while and concentrate on morphology. I got a book on the history of the English language and the contribution of other languages to English. This method helped him a great deal and he learnt to spell and read much faster, as the background of history helped his memory. Children with dyslexia struggle with executive functions, which is why, for instance, planning is so hard for them. We start working with them from the time they are very young and focus on their executive functions and soft skills. We don't wait till they are teenagers. Friendships, especially, are a very big area of concern. A long time ago, I used to teach a child who had some difficulties—partially SLD, but also other kinds of difficulties with sensory integration. She used to attend a regular school and they were good with her. But I went in there one day during the lunch break and she was sitting alone and eating. The other kids didn't know who I was. I went up and asked them, 'Why is that girl sitting by herself?' They said, 'Aunty, she doesn't know how to talk.' These children may not have read enough—they may not have heard of Harry Potter. They may not be clued into things that other children are familiar with and talk about easily. This gives us an idea of what we should do as special educators. We need to teach children to carry on a conversation. This has to be taught formally. I always made it a point to do so. I always told the parents that they have to cooperate; I can only help academically. The parents would help me out. I would tell them how to carry on a conversation around the dinner table.

What is a conversation? Most people don't think about it. It comes naturally. So, those kinds of things have to be taught. This sort of hands-on teaching is a part of SLD in some cases. One thing I like to do is to teach the parents to be advocates. That is very important, so parents can support each other better. Parent groups are also important. We teach them how to talk about their child with pride and acceptance. Parents tend to be self-conscious about their children. This shouldn't be the case. The first question I ask parents usually is, 'What do you like about your child? What can they do?' But they generally can't answer. I tell them, don't tell me what they can't do.

Srilata: How do you, as a special educator, work with parents of children with SLD?

Nirmala: It is difficult for the parent emotionally, of course. As part of our training as special educators, we need to be taught to help the parents to see things differently. Sometimes parents ask me things like, 'How do I prioritise things so I can help my child?' I always sit with the parents and with the child, if they are older, so they feel a part of things. I really enjoy that. One child said, 'I need time to go to the gym!' So, it is important to factor all that in.

Parents should get the support of the rest of the family, including the extended family. They always say they feel lonely.

I sometimes tell husbands that they should make sure their mothers understand the issue if it is a joint family. I often ask, 'May I speak to others in your family?' Once, a mother from a joint family said she was hardly ever able to leave the kitchen. She asked me, 'What do I do? I can't help my child.' I told her we would have to find a teacher for the child. That was the only way. We have to look at what is possible for the family. There is no one ideal solution.

Srilata: Describe for me some of the high points of your work as a special educator. Did your early life point you to this in some way?

Nirmala: I can't think of a life without this. I can't ever retire! It is a part of my life. When I was in school, people thought I was not a good enough student. I could never be taught. I had to learn on my own. I used to question the ones who came first in class: 'How do you learn?' They would say, 'We don't read the whole chapter.' I never knew how to game the system. There was a girl in my class who I used to write essays for every day. Later, I realised that perhaps she didn't know how to write at all! We all have learning issues! The borders are very thin. My sisters were all brilliant. Once I went to college, I was fine.

As for the high points—I used to have back-to-back classes. One day, I had a splitting headache and my blood pressure was high. So, I told this child, 'Look, today I have a bad headache. Normally, I smile when I teach. But today if I don't smile, don't think I am angry with you.' As he was leaving, he told the child who was waiting to come in not to trouble me since I had a headache! Once, a child I was teaching came from home carrying a small bag. After class, he said, 'I am going to stay here today.' He said he had a fight with his mother. So, he had packed and was ready to stay over! I could just think—my God, what trust he has! I told him that it didn't work that way. When I called his mother, she said she had no idea but yes, they had had a fight.

Another child who I had been teaching since he was four was a very restless sort of chap. So, I used to put him on my lap and teach him. Later, when he was about nineteen or so, he visited me and said, 'Nirmala aunty, can I sit on your lap?'

Another child had a lot of difficulty writing. I used to teach her. Later, when she was all set to get married, she sent me her wedding invitation. She had written out the address in her own hand. She said, 'Yours was the only address I wrote out personally because you were the one who taught me.'

Srilata: What qualities should a special educator have?

Nirmala: Humanity. And a balance between professionalism and the personal touch. Professional enough so you know what you are doing, so the parents trust you. At the same time, you should be open enough for them to feel free to talk to you. You have to earn their trust and respect, and maintain confidentiality. You should be able to listen to their story without being judgemental. You should also not be too involved with them. You shouldn't become 'friends', start visiting them. Then you can't be professional. You can't tell them certain things frankly then. But emotional connection is important—just not in the sense of becoming their friends. You should be a place that they are going to outside of themselves.

Srilata: Have you ever felt drained by your work?

Nirmala: At certain times, yes. What I do is, I protect myself before I start. I meditate, say a prayer, give myself time. I also keep aside time to do other things—care for my own children, cooking, etc.

When with the children, your focus has to be very sharp at all times. You have to watch them. I can't get up and go away when I am assessing them. I have to be physically present at all times. So, that one hour when you teach them is very intense. I used to teach from 3 p.m. to 7 p.m. So, it is a strain.

You have to protect yourself. You should not get too attached to the child, because then every single thing will affect you. Whatever you can do, you do. One child who was autistic was seven when he came to me. Sometimes, he would start screaming in the night, and the mother would call me. At such times, I couldn't say, 'I am sorry, I can't help.' So, I would call the child and speak to him. We discovered that whenever there was drilling going on in the road, he would react to that. So, we can't cut off from our students. But again, we have to protect ourselves.

Srilata: Did your work impact the way you brought up your own children?

Nirmala: Yes, one very happy thing that happened was that because of my profession, my children were sensitised to these issues at a very early age, particularly because I took classes at home. I used to have a room outside where I would teach the children. While my children were busy with their homework, I would teach my students. Then my children would like to come out and play with my students after they were done. They formed their own methods of communication. I never told my children anything—they have accepted differences in a natural way; there was no need to teach them anything. When my older son was in the first standard, he said to me, 'There is a child in my class who speaks very differently. All the children laugh, but I don't laugh. You need to come and see him.' I said I would try and talk to the child's mother.

When I started speaking to the child's mother, it turned out that the child had a cleft palate. So, my children used to identify these issues.

I hope this will help them throughout their lives. It has also taught them to be different from others. I never used to ask them about their marks or grades. I only said, 'Do better next time.' Our relatives used to tell me, 'Look, if you do this kind of work, your children will turn out like those children. Or they will start to copy them.' I would say, 'No, they will help those children.'

One Person *Can* Make a Difference

A Conversation with Namita Jacob

> Namita Jacob is currently the director of Chetana Trust,
> which designs storybooks for children with just about any
> kind of disability.

Srilata: What was it that drew you to special education?

Namita: When I started out in life, I had no particular
interest in special education. In fact, I wasn't even particularly
interested in education. The last thing I wanted to do in life
was to be a teacher. I had a completely different life plan
and kind of fell into this by chance. I was working in the
area of health. That was my primary interest—public health
and rural or community development. Health is such a large
part of what we see around us. Public health involves health
issues that can be prevented, health issues that are tied to a
sort of a lack of thinking. It's not even a lack of information.
It's more a lack of seeing yourself as someone who is able
to change your own patterns. So, that was really what I was
interested in right from my school days. And when I was in
Women's Christian College pursuing psychology, driven by
my interest in public health, I began to work in this slum
located close to our college. The idea was to work with the
Madras Corporation to clean up stagnant water. We held
a meeting in the slum and the people there told us that
the thing they really wanted was for us to help with their
children's homework. I got into it very grudgingly, recognising
that theirs was a valid request. So, though we were actually
working on nutrition and health, in between all that, for a

couple of hours every week (on Wednesdays and Fridays we were permitted to come out of college), I started to help the children with their school work. We operated out of a space in front of the headman's hut. The kids would gather there and I would randomly group them according to their size and age. We would then help with their homework. I also took some general classes in language, general knowledge, thinking, problem-solving and math. I think it was after our first or second session that the second wife of the headman (his first wife had died in childbirth) came to us, holding this very twisted, puppet-like tiny creature who was completely naked and soaking wet. She held him up from under his arms and he was all folded, like a little towelette. She then propped him up in front of the hut and said, 'Keep an eye on him, will you? If he falls down, then just prop him up again.' I was not excited at the prospect, as you can imagine! Every so often, the child would topple and I'd put him back and return to my teaching. I realised at some point that the child was always looking straight at me.

Srilata: How old was the child?

Namita: He was three. I figured he was looking straight at me for balance. What I didn't realise was that he was listening. At some point, I got irritated. In under an hour, I had had to pick him and prop him up so many times! So, finally, I picked him up gingerly, like he was some kind of rag doll, and put him down close to where I was. Next to him, between him and me, there was this group of really tiny kids. We were working on simple numbers. And when I do number concepts, I do quantities. So, I was doing addition, subtraction, etc. The children used to call me kuchi akka (stick elder sister) because I used sticks plucked from a drumstick tree to teach them. I had these bunches of sticks and went about making circles, telling them some random story and shifting the sticks from one point to another. The children had to point to the right answer. At some point, I did a three-step problem. The children were pointing to what they thought was the answer, discussing it amongst themselves and so on. Suddenly, I looked at the headman's child and said, '*Yennada intha pasanga ippadi pandraanga?* (What is going on? Why are these children acting like this?)' And he was grinning, you know, from ear to ear. And he was looking at the correct answer! And I was like, see, he knows! What the hell is going on? Was that a mere accident? I said to the kids, '*Pathya, avanukku theriyum, unakku theriyuma? Neenga nalla yosichu elaarum correct answer sollanum.* (Did you see that? He knows the answer. Do you? You have to think properly and come up with the right answer.)' After that, I made it part of the game to always ask the headman's child, '*Dei, nee sollu, da, Suresh, enna?* (Suresh, go ahead and tell us what the answer is.)' And he would always look at the right answer! At some point, I called a halt to this game, went over to him and tested him properly. And he looked at all the right answers! He was three years old. I just couldn't sleep that night. I wondered about the point of all my schooling and college education. What was the point, really, when all my assumptions had been so thoroughly, absolutely, completely wrong? I was mortified. I did some research and learnt that the child's condition was classified under 'abnormal psychology'. Just think of the words associated with things! It is 'abnormal psychology', it is 'atypical development'. And we didn't get to any of this until year three in college. Even my faculty couldn't come up with any responses beyond the usual expressions of pity and sympathy. You know, the focus is on everything that is *wrong* with the person. I went searching for services. This was in the 1980s. Vidya Sagar had just been established in Chennai. Everywhere else I went, people would point me towards mental retardation. There was just that one category! I went to two or three institutions, which I will not name, and was horrified. In my city, in times I thought of as modern ... The conditions there for children were horrific. I took the headman's wife, the stepmother of that child, to one of those places (she would have been happy to be rid of him). But even she took one look at the place, came out looking really angry and said, 'I will not do this to anybody. Which idiot would place their child here? I don't belong to that category of human beings!' And she then proceeded to scold me roundly. I had to tell her that I had no idea the place would turn out to be this bad. By the time I found Vidya Sagar, that child had passed away. And it has always been a thought in my mind—because it was so sudden—whether he was allowed to die. Was it a case of selective neglect? Was it convenience? I don't think they would have actually done something to him, but maybe it was a cold, a cough or a fever and maybe he was allowed to go. He was just three and a half ...

The six months I knew this child ended up changing my life. I felt like I owed it to him to figure out how to do better by children with such challenges. There *had* to be other options. This couldn't be the only one. After that, I was unstoppable. You learn, you go seeking places and people, you find them ... you have to keep learning. So, if you look at my preparation and trajectory, I have jumped from working with one disability to another. I started with cerebral palsy because of that child, and went on to intellectual impairment and learning disabilities, because that was the field in which I volunteered. Alpha to Omega was just being established at the time. One year into their programme, I joined as a volunteer and stayed on as a teacher. I wanted to study learning disabilities and I signed up for various courses where they dealt with slow learning, intellectual impairments, etc. I began seeing that it had nothing to do with impairment. It had everything to do with us. Lalita (from Alpha to Omega) was slowly nudging me into becoming a teacher, even though I was still resisting the idea. I kept saying, 'I don't like teaching. I will be very bored. I will design aids. I will do all the surrounding stuff, but don't make me teach. I don't like kids.' And Lalita would draw me in, ask me to help her out with stuff. She assigned one child to me—a tiny plum of a sweetheart. He was in standard four—had never passed anything—although they really wanted him to be still sitting in standard three. He had done standard three twice already. They had pushed him up with many threats and what not. The parents were saying if he cannot get through his papers this year, we will need to reconsider this whole thing. So, he was given to me along with a set of strategies that I didn't totally understand. I was still learning and reading up. I followed some of them even though I thought it was nonsense—you know, all these gimmicky things: bounce the ball this way, that way and arrange the alphabets and do this and that. I had to get through that one hour with him and between Lalita and I, we used to develop this hour-long plan. But gradually, this child, who had never scored above thirty, began to score in the sixties and seventies. He made that leap from 'Will I pass, will I pass, will I pass, will I fail?' to 'Am I going to make it to a first class?' That was such a surprise. In three months, in just three months, he had managed this. And for the past four–five years that poor kid had been struggling. The point is that the education he had received was idiotic, the method was idiotic and we didn't see it. I felt I needed to do something about this. That's when I took up Special Education professionally.

Srilata: Tell me about Chetana. Who is it meant for?

Namita: I believe very strongly that if you see a problem and it bothers you, you have an obligation to try and address it, especially as someone who has been educated. The question always is, 'How can one person make a difference?' Special education teaches you that one person *can* make a difference. Even if it is one life you change, that's a big deal in itself. I do believe that you need an organisation, you need something bigger than just focusing on a kid. It has to be everything that surrounds a child. I realised I didn't fit very well anywhere. I thought perhaps the best thing I could do was to remain outside and provide support from there. Chetana started because I was frustrated about various things at that time. One frustration was about the absence of storybooks for blind children. I had been working with visually impaired kids and was once sent a child from the Blind School. Her teachers sent her to me with the question: Is she retarded? The other common assumption, of course, is if the child is not retarded then the problem must lie with the parents. There are only these two options. The third option, 'You guys don't know how to teach', is on nobody's radar.

Here they are, located inside a special education environment, and exhibiting this kind of mindset! I spoke to this child and it was clear to me that she was totally brilliant, that she had a flair for language. She could speak, she could hear and pick up all sorts of things! Her capacity and range were incredible. She switched between multiple languages during our conversation. Listening to her, looking at her, I could only think, 'Which teacher looked at you and thought you were retarded?' She had scored above 70 per cent in every subject and had failed in Braille! I had to make very small adjustments to help her. I helped her find ways in which she could arrange and organise her body and her brain to do well. And I wanted her to practise not with these stupid Braille books they were giving—the 'A' page was full of 'A's, the 'B' page was full of 'B's, and so on. This child was not three years old! Actually, they shouldn't have been giving this to a three-year-old either, let alone an older child at that level. I wanted to offer her storybooks. I asked her, 'What storybooks do you have in your library?' She said there were none. 'What storybooks do you have at home?' I asked. She said she had none at home either. 'What storybooks have you read?' I asked. She had never read a storybook! She had only *heard* of them! I thought of it as an insult—to hand her a book that was created for a little child. So, I went hunting. I went to the School for the Blind, I went everywhere, but drew a blank! There was nothing ...

I had a friend, Shanti, whose daughter, Sumi, had always been into books. I was sitting in my living room with her one day and she went, 'Okay, I'll try to do it. I will make storybooks for blind children.' So, we talked about it and that's how it all started. We asked ourselves what were the things that needed to be adjusted when it came to storybooks for blind children and we went about doing it.

I used to work with multiple schools as their consultant. Each school hired me for one or the other of my skillset. At Vidya Sagar, I was hired for early intervention and working with deaf children. There were three of them at the time— three students who had hearing impairment in addition to cerebral palsy. And I was having great fun working with them. One was very tiny. One was older and the third one was an adult. I would work on developing teaching material, work with speech centres and so on. And then I would also work with the babies. After about a week or ten days, maybe a little longer, I was talking with the director when I asked her, 'So who is working with the VI (visually impaired) kids?' And she went, 'What VI kids? We only have one child, Akash. That fellow you're already helping.' Which was true. I was helping him. I said, 'No, no, he is blind. But what about kids with low vision?' She said, 'We don't have anyone like that. There's that one fellow with one eye; are you talking about him?' I said, 'No, no, in every class, there are children with low vision.'

'You mean children with a squint?'

I said, 'No, I mean children with low vision.'

She said, 'No, what are you talking about?'

I said to her, 'How can you not see it?'

And she responded, 'All you people go abroad and super specialise. You come back, and all you see is disability and impairment.'

I thought to myself, 'That's not fair. That is not true. How can she say that? I have to prove it to her. There are children with low vision and other forms of VI in here.' So, I said, 'Alright. Pick any class in this school and I will tell you how many children there are who I think have vision impairment. I will take them to Sankara Nethralaya. I will get them assessed. And then you'll get an objective opinion.' We did that and sure enough, of course, those children had visual impairments!

The director was really upset and she said, 'We have to fix this. We need to have the whole school assessed.' And then came the problem. Because I wanted the entire school assessed as well but it wasn't going to be easy ... We couldn't just name, identify and then, nothing. For them to diagnose and say this child has this part of his system impaired, for them to say, 'You have optic nerve atrophy' or 'You have retinopathy' ... that is identification. That, they can do. But what do you do about it afterwards? And also, I had gone through that first set of appointments and I could see that neither ophthalmologists nor optometrists nor those clinics had the capacity, the tools or the perspective required to assess these children. When you go in for an eye exam, there are two parts to it. One part where they will dilate and look inside your eye, but also another part where they ask you to read things, to respond, which is not easy with our kids. It's not impossible, but it's not easy. And if you don't know the strategy, it's impossible. They don't have a chair that works for our children. If you don't sit right, I am not going to ask you to stand on tip-toe on one foot and read the eye chart. And they think the smallest line you read is really an indication of your vision. So, if you do the same to my child and he is balancing on a chair like this, he is not going to read the line that he can actually read. There were so many things. How do you ask a question of a child who only has one-word answers to give? He can only say, 'Yes.' How do you ask the question if your Braille is not going to work? There was another problem too ... the doctors were so overwhelmed on seeing these kids. They did not want to trouble them any further. They did not want them to make the effort to read a chart, to go to all that trouble! But what they didn't see was that these kids are actually studying and so of course they can read a chart. And also, their vision needs to be assessed like any other child! Their attitude was, 'Let's not trouble them. They can be fitted with glasses later. That's alright. This much vision is good enough for them.' So, we really had to think of another approach altogether. They were fully qualified professionals but did not have the skills to assess these kids. It was obvious that if you really wanted to do this right, you were going to have to do multiple things. You were going to have to create something for parents, you were going to have to create something for the teachers. You were going to have to create something for the older children so they could understand their own situation. You were going to have to create something for doctors, for ophthalmologists. You were going to have to create a referral framework. It was bigger than just saying, 'Okay, test all the children in the school and give them glasses.' That wasn't going to fix anything. Also, there was no point in saying we will assess these kids first and then think about it. I can't function like that. For me, that's playing dirty. You don't do that. You don't identify a whole bunch of children and then just leave them hanging while you think of the next step. I wanted to do it properly. Because I knew that if, in fact, I wanted to change systems, I would have to standardise the documentation around it. I would have to publish it or present it to a medical fraternity so they would be convinced that they had to do something about it. I wanted to get them all assessed, but I didn't want to compromise on the process, because I felt the process would allow us to create valid systems here.

Nobody was willing to take me up. I asked Sankara Nethralaya, I asked anyone and everyone but nobody wanted to get involved with something that was so effortful. They wanted funding before they would actually start. I felt one must start right away since there was a problem. You know, if I didn't know there was this problem, I wouldn't have minded, but now I knew. It was not just an academic question.

Srilata: Every day is precious. It matters for the child.

Namita: Yes, it's a day lost. When I was talking about this, everyone kept saying to me, 'Start an NGO.' Again, just like teaching, the last thing I ever wanted to do with my life was to deal with starting this and that. Then, Shanti, Anil (my husband) and my dad said, 'Let's form a trust.' My dad, Anil and I decided to put in 30 per cent from our income. And that was enough for me to get started. I was not looking to be paid. I just wanted the expenses covered. Also, it helped to have a trust when you were working with parents and needed permissions. Chetana was a way to do the work that nobody else was willing to take up.

Srilata: Do you still continue to work with assessments of children?

Namita: As far as assessments of children in schools is concerned, I have distanced myself from that a bit. Schools are trained now and can always come to me when they have questions, when they want to discuss their protocols or need some tools. It is now all part of the curriculum, it's now in the policy, it's in the school of optometry, it's in Sankara Nethralaya. We have MPhil students, we have PhD students. We have vision centres set up. Yes, I continue to stay associated and available, but that's it. They all run independently. It took us ten years to get to that point. Now what we do is maintenance. Once in two years we run a training week where people come in. Chetana has partnered with Vidya Sagar to run the 'I Count' training programme—'I Count' as in 'eye counts', or my vision, my eyes count, but also I as a person count. When you do the math, it's shocking. 66 per cent of the children we assessed had a vision impairment that was unidentified. All these children had neurological impediments.

Srilata: And nobody had identified that?

Namita: Some of them had been assessed and the problem had been identified, but they had not received any follow-up interventions. But many of them were being diagnosed for the first time.

Srilata: Right ...

Namita: Even things like, 'He just needs to be fitted with glasses.' Or, 'It is just a case of refractive error.' And these children really need to see well. They can't move. They can't talk. So, if you don't even bother to correct their vision, then it is so difficult. Also, it is important to ask, 'Correct for what? For what distance? For what purpose? To see what?'

Srilata: They may not go out into the world, but they may need to read off a screen ...

Namita: Correct. Or they may not be looking at screens, but they may want to see your face, your expressions, they may want to see the distance they can't get to. When you go to ophthalmologists these days, they will ask you, 'Do you spend more time reading print or reading off a computer screen?' Why do they ask you that question? Because it's distance. Right? It's distance and science. It helps make a decision about correction. Who asks my kids what they want to see? They simply declare, 'This dioptre equals this correction.' It's a mathematical formula that assumes a certain way of living and the importance of seeing something specific that may not be important to my kid at all. So, a lot of it is perspective.

Srilata: Does the same thing hold for hearing-impaired children with cerebral palsy as well? That they are not identified, or that the intervention is not proper ...

Namita: We haven't started on that yet ...

Srilata: I was thinking of how we sometimes deal with elderly people. We don't properly identify issues because we tell ourselves they are old in any case and don't really need the intervention.

Namita: Yes. And then you correct it and you *see* the difference and you think, 'Oh, my God! It was such a small step. Why didn't I do it before?'

So now we have made it a regular practice—once a year we do a school-wide screening and every year we have caught developing cataracts. You see, these kids are on medications too. Many of them have the disability because of other underlying issues.

My college notes on cerebral palsy from the 1990s clearly say that 75 per cent of children with this condition will also have a vision impairment. The research dates back to the 1970s. So, it's not an unknown factor. But we don't know what to do with it. If I look at visual impairment in a typical developing population versus visual impairment in a population with neurological impediments, more than half of the latter is going to have to have a visual impairment. But what we do is we ignore this big group and focus on the typical group, where about 30 per cent of the children are likely to require spectacles. We have completely ignored the biggest group that is most likely to require correction, support and intervention.

The conversation is now out there and a lot of these places now have many of the tools we developed, much of the materials we have developed. We just put everything we develop up on our website or we give it out for free during training. So, we started out of that frustration and that need. And a lot of people have asked me, 'How do you scale up?' But I don't feel any obligation to scale up. I think the way we scale up is to share knowledge and other people should then do their job. They are free to copy our process. You want me to come and help you? I will come, but you do the work.

Srilata: Tell me about the people who volunteer with Chetana.

Namita: A lot of people who volunteer with us tend to be people who are confused about their lives, people going through depression, people going through mental illness. I have, as a volunteer, someone who is terminally ill. The act of giving back, the act of doing something that will impact another person's life, is a healing.

I don't agree when people tell me, 'Oh, you must be such a nice person.' What I'm doing is, in fact, the most selfish thing you can do with your life. I wake up every day saying, 'What am I going to do?' Every night I have something to celebrate. How many people have jobs like that? And it is so valuable also because there's no money in it. So, for me, it is about remaining a volunteer service. Chetana is about helping people understand that they can learn how to work in this field. People come up to me and say, '*Yenakku ithu pathi theriyille* (I don't know about this field)'. They say, 'I would love to work in this place. I know how to draw, to write scripts ... but I don't know anything about this.' I say to them, 'Guess what? You can learn!' You know, it isn't impossible. You don't even need to be literate; you just need to have common sense. There's nothing difficult about it. I even invite children with disabilities to work with us. I invite anyone who has an interest to work with us. There's no pre-qualification. The only thing I ask for is that you are consistent. You can't commit to something and run away, so you take that decision. If you aren't able to do it, then I'll do it. So, my volunteers learn sign language because when students or colleagues come in and ask, 'Who is there to support the deaf, blind or visual impaired?' I expect everyone in the room to know how to respond and how to be supportive.

Chetana is to sense or become aware of. It can also be about creating awareness, spreading awareness and I feel it's both that we need to do. We need to develop an understanding of what is missing, figure out that pathway and then follow through. We have now moved into creating a library as a way, both of learning as well as providing. We have created a simple curriculum because we realised that we had children who could, for example, read Braille and understand but had no real world understanding of some objects. They would ask, '*Yennakka ithu?* (What is this, akka?)'. And I can't tell you how many children I have come across like that. If I were to tell these kids, 'Unzip your bag,' they would. But if gave them my bag and said, 'Unzip my bag' and the zip were oriented differently, they don't know how to tackle it. They may look like they are independent, but they have zero problem-solving skills. That's horrible! So much depends on their figuring this stuff out. Even kids from the same school, for example, there will be kids who have figured it out and those who haven't. The kids who were not taught—they are thinkers with their fingers. The difference between them and the other kids is like night and day.

Srilata: So, does this happen only with children who are blind at birth or also with children who have lost their vision when young?

Namita: We've seen it with kids with low vision as well. It is to do with a complete lack of exposure. So, if you give them a very simple image, like circles and squares, or a very nice Braille that is easy to see, yes. But if you give them an image that's a little less clear, then that internal voice, the

voice that drives you to make an effort—it doesn't exist. They
will simply say, 'I can't see.' That's that. No one has given
these kids any strategies. So, they will look at a page and
say, 'I can't see.' And then if I give them a strategy and say,
'Can you find something of a different colour in this one?'
'Yes.' 'Can you put your finger on it?' 'Yes.' 'Can you come
close to it now and look at it and tell me what you think it
is?' They will then name the thing. Where is the, 'I can't see?'
You can see! You just haven't tried, no? And that 'can't see'
comes from that. So, in my mind it's these two things. There's
no internal perception of yourself as someone who can use
your hands to learn and zero strategy. So then you remain
dependent on someone. What we realised with our books is
that we need to have multiple versions. So, you have ones
with simple text, simple images. You've simple text, complex
images. You have complex text, simple images, or complex
text, complex images. You need all these options. You have
to cater to all reading levels. And the language has to be kept
really simple and illustrations have to be used to support
the language ... The reading levels of a lot of our deaf kids
and other kids isn't very high. And the effort to read is so
much that they are not able to enjoy the story, but if I tell
them a story, they will enjoy it. But if you ask them to read
that book, it's too much. Many things about it make it too
much. It's too many pages. Even if it's two, three lines on a
page, they look at a book this thick and they hesitate. Making
the text-size bigger really helps. We chunk information in a
certain way so that it helps comprehension. We reduced the
repetitiveness. The illustrations we use tell a story too. So,
they can just look at the pictures and get the whole story.
They can access a book at their social, emotional, cognitive
level, at their language level and at their picture level.

The Skill to Listen to Their Silences

A Conversation with Nandini Santhanam

Nandini Santhanam is the founder-director of The Lotus Foundation, a learning centre for people on the autism spectrum.

Srilata: Tell me about yourself. What led you to this field?

Nandini: My mother was schizophrenic. My father worked for the Reserve Bank. Following his retirement, they came down to Chennai. At the age of sixty-seven, he had severe seizures lasting many days. Doctors brought him around but he suffered memory loss and was diagnosed with autism. It was most unusual. His entire character and temperament, his very perspective was transformed. So, autism became my calling. After my father's diagnosis, my parents lived a rich and fulfilling life for fourteen years, managing what was most important to them. I happen to be an only child. I started to observe that my parents were now living a far more independent life (following my father's autism diagnosis) than when my father was still in service. I found this most interesting.

Srilata: How did this happen?

Nandini: I don't know. It was their process entirely and it liberated me from any day-to-day caregiving. They got to know their neighbours, made friends and supported each other. This was very effective socially. They had one group of friends to walk with, another group to discuss their ailments or go to the hospital with. I was drawn to autism, to people with autism. This was back in 1994. I had never heard of the term prior to that. I started to train in the field. I used to work broadly in the area of technology. I now decided to pursue psychology. I felt that would give me an insight into autism. I completed a masters in the subject and followed it up with some training in special education. I had different options open to me. I could, for instance, work with children who had learning disabilities or were autistic. Eventually, I ended up working for We-Excel, an educational trust based in Chennai committed to helping people with special needs. I was with them for ten years, heading their remedial unit. I would meet three to five sets of parents every day. These meetings gave rise to a lot of questions within me. What were we doing with human beings? We were teaching them to write, read, learn. But we didn't know what the students knew. We were merely teaching the children the tools and the methods that would allow them to fit in! I gave up my job at We-Excel and set up The Lotus Foundation. I discarded everything I knew. Life became beautiful after that. My head was full of new ideas, questions and thoughts. Why was autism so prevalent now? We had always known 'slow' people but autism wasn't about that because these kids were very smart. So, I decided to specialise in autism. I wrote up a whole new curriculum that would suit my needs. For eight years, I didn't talk to anybody about it. Two years ago, I submitted this curriculum for a conference in which I was required to make a presentation. It was published. My mentor and co-founder, Vijay, has travelled all over India, lecturing and conducting workshops, on new ways of looking at autism.

Srilata: What are some of these new ways of looking at autism?

Nandini: I did not have a theory I was trying to prove. I was just asking for answers. Why is the spirit or consciousness so deep, so hidden? If your consciousness and mine are the same, why are you and I not alike? I came to this beautiful idea called law of attraction: like attracts like. I applied that to what I knew about autism. I found that at a deep level, these children and I are alike—at the deepest spiritual level. But we have a different exterior. Then I began to ask questions about pre-birth intentions. What happens when you decide to be an autistic person, when you decide to choose this life? That gave me a lot of answers. All of us want something. We want to do something. We basically want to be happy with who we are. If our only purpose is to be happy as this person, you can be happy. These days we discard old technology for new; the same thing happens to humans too. We go out of this world and come back to it. We shed our old bodies; we upgrade ourselves. These children can speak but have decided not to. They have chosen not to. What kind of *vairagyam* or destiny is that, to not speak at all, all your life? What drives these children to withhold speech? Are they not communicating? They are! What language are they using? This question led me to try and communicate with them. I have, in the last two years, developed the skill to listen to their silences. This has come after a lot of inner work. It is no rocket science. This work has helped me make sense of the children's inner lives. A child either gives me the permission to understand them or not. Teenagers with autism have some difficulty during puberty. They explain it to the world in their own way but the world doesn't pay attention, doesn't give them that time. All that these children may require is a break, a day of silence, a day of no activity which too is a kind of activity. They may take time to transition. They may grow aggressive. We try to treat them with psychiatric drugs, we beat them up, we tie them up. We try to fit a beautiful round peg into a square hole. That doesn't work. The nature of autism is that it is not curable. How many ever years of therapy you give people with autism, it is you who has to change. Autistic people possess strong will. They wish to share with the world ideas of the highest nature, of sheer joy. Everybody is free to be who they are. If I could take the liberty to be who I am, wouldn't that be the most beautiful thing? What is stopping me? It is only my thoughts.

The Child Is a Person First

An Interview with Poonam Natarajan

Poonam Natarajan, a parent of a child with high support needs, founded Vidya Sagar in 1985, in Chennai. It is well known for its range of services for people with intellectual and developmental disabilities. She also served as chairperson, National Trust for Persons with Autism, Cerebral Palsy, Intellectual Disability and Multiple Disability. This is a statutory body under the Ministry of Social Justice and Empowerment, Government of India.

Srilata: You started Vidya Sagar primarily because you were looking for a place for your son, Ishwar. In the absence of state support for persons with disabilities, many parents fall back on their own solutions. Some of these 'solutions' prove to be enabling for others in similar situations. While this is also exciting at a certain level, it isn't easy and it isn't fair. How do you feel about this?

Poonam: Vidya Sagar turns thirty-seven in 2022. We started on 15 March 1985. Yes, it started with my son Ishwar, and it has been an exciting journey, where each student has helped to create new learnings and pathways.

In the beginning, setting up services seemed like an almost impossible task. There was no roadmap for the technical expertise, the team, the infrastructure, the funding needed. It all depended on one's own creative expertise. However, we received amazing support from the community and the people around. The work absorbed me completely; it showed me my own strengths and the power of the collective. Many, many people participated in putting the pieces together to create what is Vidya Sagar today. Yes, in the process, the boundaries between my personal and professional life have become fuzzy and blurred—that's my art of living now!

Srilata: Have attitudes towards disability changed in this country?

Poonam: Yes, they have. Many services for the disabled in the country have been started by parents. In a way, this has also helped to demonstrate different models of service delivery. There has been a paradigm shift in the understanding of disability. We have moved on from the earlier medical and charity models to the social, development and human rights models. The state, however, has been slow to recognise these changes and disability remains a very low priority. In fact, it is sad to see state funding being reduced even in the government's own projects, like inclusive education, early intervention or even the Accessible India Campaign. There should be a disability component in all government schemes, like health, housing and insurance.

Srilata: Tell me about your son, Ishwar. What was he like? What was it like for you to have him in your life?

Poonam: Ishwar (Ishoo, as we called him) was our only child, very precious and important in our life. When we realised that he had disabilities, we tried to understand what his needs were and what we should do. Just finding that out was impossible. It led me to quit my academic pursuits, to train in the field.

Ishoo had multiple special needs and we understood that he may not be able to study and work, like many children with disabilities. Children like Ishoo are said to have a poor prognosis and, therefore, are not valued or given admission even in special schools.

Ishoo, in a way, became our guru. He taught us to look at life in many different ways. He taught us how each person is valuable and that disability is just a way of life, to be enjoyed, appreciated and lived fully.

My husband and I were classmates in the MA programme at Jawaharlal Nehru University. We had explored and understood many dimensions of marginalisation, but it was Ishoo who taught us about disability. In the beginning there was, of course, the despair and heartbreak. But as we went on over the years, we were grateful that he chose us as his parents, and took us along a path we had not imagined or planned. It is a journey which has been very fulfilling.

Srilata: Your intention when Vidya Sagar was set up was to involve and train the parents of children with disabilities as well. Did that work well? What was the basic vision behind Vidya Sagar? What did you hope to achieve?

Poonam: I first set up the centre in our garage, as a branch of The Spastic Society of India, Mumbai. That was where I trained as a special educator with Dr Mithu Alur, who founded the latter.

In those days, I felt very strongly about demystifying disability and training parents. Parents' struggle, shopping for a cure, going from one doctor to another, while their time and energy needed to be spent on training the child. Unfortunately, doctors do not know about training and management and its importance. Since there is no medical cure for disability, they are not able to advise adequately. For a parent, it is vital to understand that disability is a lifelong condition and it is only with training and practice that the child can acquire skills.

Therefore, as a parent myself, I felt training parents on

physio, speech and occupational therapy would empower the family. These interventions are generally mystified and it is assumed that only therapists can work with the child. However, therapy works only if it is regularly practised and becomes a way of life. Transferring these skills to the parent must be an essential part of the rehabilitation process.

In the beginning, my vision was really about awareness and acceptance, and creating a peer group for my son. As we grew together as a community and as children with diverse needs began to be part of our work, our vision and plans developed.

Srilata: Could you describe for me the early years of Vidya Sagar?

Poonam: The early years were heady, to say the least. It was an amazing time, a time of discovery and learning—about myself and about disability. The first and most important need was to put together a multidisciplinary team of therapists and special educators who knew the subject and were confident and liberated enough to share their knowledge with parents. I was fortunate to find wonderful people, full of creative ideas and who loved the field they had chosen, and I think, we were the best team in the world. We were flooded with children and families. In the first week itself, forty-five families came to the centre. It broke the myth of what I had repeatedly been told before I started, that families only wanted their children to be taken care of, no one wanted to be trained. Each child made us explore and look for new strategies and there was much learning. All of us also learnt from each other; it led to the development of what we called the trans-disciplinary approach. Each one of us learnt to assess a child in all areas and plan a holistic programme. We learnt to train diverse families and children, with varying resources and literacy levels.

Many children became what we called milestone children, that is, they made us develop a whole new programme, whether early intervention, an outstation programme or vocational training.

Then there was fundraising, a whole new area, where we were novices really. We have many stories of sterling community support.

Srilata: What is it like to support and teach children with varying form of disabilities, many of which are classified as profound disabilities?

Poonam: From the beginning, the policy was no 'choosing' of students. It was agreed that any family coming to our centre needed support. Therefore, we did not refuse anyone. This made doctors also refer children with multiple special needs to us, children who were earlier called severely or profoundly disabled.

It is most important to learn to think of the child as a person first. Once we do that, whatever the disability, it becomes easy to deal with. We have multi-ability students with varying special needs.

Planning holistically with the entire team, the family and the child, if she can participate, is vital. This requires us to take time, to get everyone together and set long-term and short-term goals in all areas—motor, sensory, cognition, communication, activities of daily living, socialisation and, of course, areas like nutrition and emotional well-being. Most of the goals are achieved through play and activities that can easily be done at home. The training works when parents, grandparents and siblings get excited about the activities and understand how these will help to develop a skill and achieve a goal.

Teaching children with multiple disabilities succeeds only when the staff works together when the children are not around, when they think and plan together, create all kinds of activities, think in terms of adapting toys, books and teaching-learning materials. The staff at Vidya Sagar are fantastic at this.

Srilata: A lot of people—special educators included—often hesitate to work with children who have profound or multiple disabilities. What is the work really like on a day-to-day, minute-to-minute basis?

Poonam: Yes, there is an attitudinal barrier about working with children who have high support needs. Many schools do not give admission to these children. Some professionals may also feel it is not worth it. Actually, to my mind this work is about not being able to show dramatic progress.

At Vidya Sagar, we have learnt to work and plan in a different way. The child is a person first and we celebrate even the smallest achievement. It could be as basic as learning to grasp and release an object, getting out of diapers or it could be learning to use the computer or to skate and swim. Each of these are broken down into smaller sub-tasks. So, on a day-to-day, minute-to-minute basis, one learns how to celebrate the achieving of a sub-task.

Many times, the goal may just be about supporting the parents to accept their child and find easy ways to fulfil her needs, to get family members to learn how to live with a positive state of mind and understand that each one of us is unique, with our own strengths and weaknesses. Sometimes simple solutions of caretaking can pave the way for acceptance by the family. It is also about changing one's perspective to life.

Srilata: How does disability—experiencing it first-hand or at one remove—change one's perspective?

Poonam: As a parent, my son's disability helped me change my thinking in many ways. When one travels a different path, that experience helps one look for different answers. Joy and happiness in day-to-day life actually depends on us. As parents, it is unfair to put that burden on the shoulders of our young children. As I learnt to understand every small and minute milestone in child development, it showed me nature's miracles in amazing ways.

Experiencing disability actually helps one appreciate things that one generally takes for granted. Even every day events like the sunrise and sunset become more beautiful and fill one with a sense of gratitude. You unlearn many things school conditions us with, like competing, like uniformity, like what achievement really means. Like the futility of marks and examinations and the importance of collaborating. Like understanding that disability is not an individual problem but a community issue.

Even people with disabilities need to work on a perspective while coming to terms with their weaknesses and strengths.

Srilata: It seems to me—especially from speaking to parents of children with disabilities—that one needs to do a lot of inner work to completely accept one's child for what he or she is. And I suppose this is, at some level, an ongoing journey. Can you say something about that?

Poonam: Yes, of course, it is an ongoing journey—as the child goes through different stages, so does the parent. Children are the best teachers.

There is a stigma, a sadness, a loss attached to the very concept of disability. We grieve and despair. It certainly needs work to change this deep conditioning, especially when it happens to oneself. Unless we do that work, we can never make a rehabilitation programme work.

As a mother, in the beginning I felt very low and sometimes desperate. My husband reminded me that the three of us need not drown in this experience of Ishoo having a disability. He said we also had a commitment to life, to celebrate it and to enjoy it. This perspective laid the foundation that shaped our thinking and living together.

Home for Lunch

Lakshmi Govindarajan

Lakshmi Govindarajan is a retired bank employee who used to volunteer in a centre for people with disabilities and different learning styles. She loves music and crocheting.

It was the morning of the big lunch and I was really nervous. I paced up and down the house, making sure things were in place, putting the finishing touches to the meal I had spent all morning preparing. I had to ensure now that the doors to all the bedrooms and showcases in my living room were firmly shut and that my living room was stripped bare of all things except for the dining table, the chairs and the sofa.

I host lunches quite often but this was a different sort of hosting altogether. My guests were adults with special needs and I had to approach things differently. For instance, Meena would be in a wheelchair and so I had to ensure accessibility for her. Arvind was autistic and tended to get triggered by objects that he wanted but could not get his hands on. If he set eyes on something he wanted, it was difficult, if not impossible, to distract him from that. I needed also to check for sharp edges, since I did not want any of my guests to get hurt.

There is a backstory to this lunch. Following my retirement, I had taken to volunteering at a centre for adults with special needs. I am not a trained special educator, though I have completed quite a few online courses in special education. One morning, I casually told the group from the centre that they should come home for lunch sometime. Meena was taken aback and asked me over and over whether I really meant it. She was almost in tears. I was thrown by her reaction. I learnt later that children and adults with special needs do not get to interact with families that are made up of neurotypical individuals. The only exception to this tends to be important family events. When I understood this, I made up my mind to have them all over for lunch one day.

A small note about each member of this very mixed group of individuals that I work with. Each of them has a different sort of disability. Arvind is twenty-six years old and is on the autism spectrum, despite which he is very sociable. He will not make eye contact, makes a lot of repetitive movements and talks non-stop. He is very smart and has a great memory. Meena is twenty-nine years old and has cerebral palsy. She has poor muscle coordination. She is a very cheerful girl and loves dressing up and wearing coordinated accessories. Gayathri is in her sixties. Her IQ is that of a seven- or eight-year-old. Her brain development was affected because her mother took some medication when she was pregnant with her. Gayathri is hesitant to get close to people but has become good friends with Saira, Sridhar and Meena. She really enjoys chatting with me. Saira is thirty-six and has an intellectual disability. She is the oldest of her siblings. Her father, who is now no more, treated her quite badly, as a result of which Saira stopped speaking. Over time, though, she has gained some confidence and now replies to us in monosyllables. She insists on wearing flowers in her hair every day.

Baskar is forty-nine years old and has Down's syndrome. He is the friendliest person I know and is always cheerful and full of energy. Robert is fifty and has multiple sensory and motor disabilities. The only thing he seems to want to do is to draw birds. Sridhar is forty-four years old. He too has multiple sensory and motor disabilities. He cannot hear or see well and has the IQ of a young child. He is usually very quiet.

To get all of them home was no mean task. I had asked Ashok, the auto driver who I employ on a regular basis, to pick them up in small groups. The first group comprised Sridhar, Baskar, Robert and the teacher. It took a while for them to get to my place because Baskar, who is severely claustrophobic, refused to enter the elevator. Since his speech tends to be unclear and he mumbles, it took everyone some time to understand what the problem was. When the others finally figured what his problem was, it was decided that Ashok would walk up the stairs with him, while the rest took the elevator. Ashok then went back and forth transporting the other groups and soon everyone had assembled at my place—Meena, Saira, Gayatri, Saira's mother, Sam (a volunteer), Arvind, Arvind's mother and grandmother, Sridhar, Baskar, Basker's mother, Robert and the teacher.

Baskar was perhaps the most excited of the lot. He went about shaking hands with everyone and did what he liked best—praying for all of us and 'blessing' us irrespective of how old we were, the way he sees his pastor do at church. The others were quite shy because they were in an unfamiliar place. But Baskar was in his element. He went around taking photos with his make-believe camera, which was, essentially, a handkerchief folded into the shape of a mobile phone.

The teacher who had accompanied them had planned many activities for the group. As soon as I had finished serving out the juice, she got them to sing in turns. Most of them positioned their hands as a kind of pretend-microphone. But Baskar decided to use a pen instead for this purpose! They sang their favourite songs without any inhibition.

It was 1 p.m.—time for lunch. With the exception of Arvind, none of them knew how to read time. But their body clocks worked perfectly and they whipped out their water bottles in readiness for lunch! I had, at first, contemplated ordering all the food but Meena had insisted that I cook, saying she wanted to savour my cooking. I had prepared lunch keeping in mind the favourite dishes of the group. Sridhar would always go on about my *bisi bele bath*, a spicy flavoured rice, and so I just *had* to make that for him. Saira and Meena loved vegetable pulav so I had prepared that as well. Gayathri, Robert, Basker and Sridhar were usually happy eating anything, so I did not have to worry about them.

Saira's mother, Meena's mother, the teacher, my house-help and I pre-served all the food onto the plates. Each plate had a serving of the bisi bele bath, chips, pulav, raitha, potato and peas sabzi, curd rice, pickle and salad. We handed these plates out one by one. Sam and I then stood by, ready to give anyone who asked for it, a second helping. This wasn't easy because while Gayathri, Sridhar and Meena know exactly when they have had enough and are able to say so; the rest have difficulty communicating this. What complicated this task even more was the fact that Baskar and Arvind intensely disapprove of people who waste food, forcing both themselves and others to eat everything on their plates. We got through this one way or the other and then it was time for desert— vermicelli kheer.

With the meal done and everything put away, it was time for some dancing. We put on the music and soon, Sam was dancing away and the rest were on their own. Saira and Gayathri alone did not join in. Saira seemed to want to relax. Gayathri was clearly awkward and shy about dancing in her sari, which she did not want to come undone.

Soon, it was time for them to leave and Ashok was once again pressed into service.

As I have already said, I have guests over all the time and love cooking for them. But this was a different sort of cooking and hosting. For a start, I had grown especially attached to and fond of these guests. It bothered me that this was perhaps the first time they had been invited to lunch by someone like me from a family of neurotypical or 'normal' people. For my part, it meant that I had to be especially careful about the ingredients I used in the food. I had to be careful about how much spice I used, for instance, because I didn't want any of them falling ill. Some of them also had certain dietary restrictions and were in a fragile state of health. Access had to be ensured, as well as a safe environment. These guests, unlike other guests of mine, did not hesitate to say just what they thought about my cooking! And I really liked that about them. Ever since, I have had them all home for lunch at least twice a year.

Reflections of a Special Educator

Anuradha Shyam

Anuradha Shyam has worked as a special educator for ten years, interacting and learning with a wide range of students. Currently based in Bengaluru, her life revolves around her family and their pet dog.

A MIRROR CALLED RADHIKA

Radhika walked into the classroom as I waited with an air of expectancy tinged with the trepidation of a novice. She was my first student, assigned a week after I had been certified as a special educator. There was a storm of defiance in her eyes. Her limbs darted everywhere. Alphabet blocks and hand puppets sailed across the room in abandon. A bloodcurdling scream arose from the depth of her being as she opened the door and hurtled down the corridor. Our session was over, even before it had started. Triumphant, she grinned, claiming victory over my collapsing facade of professionalism. Parents waiting with their children and colleagues exchanged smiles. Mortified, I headed back to the room.

For the next six sessions, this ritual was followed with meticulous precision. Radhika's methods may have been varied but her intent was clear—she was neither going to be cajoled nor coerced into a session. The frustration of not being able to connect with my student, coupled with an impatience to prove myself, only compounded my growing sense of despair. Over the next few days, I read extensively and conferred with colleagues, seeking their advice. All of this stemmed from a self-imposed anxiety; I had excelled in the course and what

I was experiencing now was a hard blow to my pride. The seventh day I was to meet Radhika, I decided would be our last. I was going to request for a change of student.

As she walked in that day, an idea flashed through my mind. Without thinking twice, I started to run around the room, hands flaying, knocking down everything in my path. I jumped up and down, made faces that mirrored Radhika's and rendered her version of a war cry. This entire charade lasted under a minute. The look on my student's face was invaluable. It was as though she was seeing me for the first time. Transfixed, she walked quietly towards the chair and sat down, looking at me with a newfound respect. Our first session had begun.

Twelve years have passed but what Radhika taught me that day about teaching is still fresh in my mind. Teaching happens when a teacher is willing to lay down the armour of intellectual and professional pride, and meet the student at the point where the student is willing to be met. As educators, and certainly as special educators, we need to train in theoretical knowledge to prepare for what we can bring to the classroom; however, unless we allow experience and intuition to also guide how we teach, we will not be able to even reach the students we are meant to teach. Accepting that we are in a space of not knowing keeps us receptive to the challenges that each student brings. From Radhika I learnt that disability is not apart from life. It is an expression of it. As Radhika's teacher, I was in partnership with her; every step she took towards realising her potential mirrored my own growth and evolution.

～

LOVE IN HOLDING ON, LOVE IN LETTING GO

In the course of my work as a special educator, I have sometimes met parents who have redefined for me notions of courage and love. Seema, a parent of a young adult with autism, was one such parent. She told me one day about how she had tackled the issue of her grown-up son soiling himself.

He had flatly refused to clean himself and was resistant to all help. In utter exasperation, Seema, who had tried many a strategy, decided to adopt a new one. From then on, she decided, no one in the family would assist him when it came to changing clothes. He would have to do so himself. The first week, his resistance to personal hygiene only seemed to grow stronger. For the next two weeks, they had to live with a human stink bomb. Neighbours stopped dropping by, Seema's extended family beseeched her to drop this strategy, and her son became house-bound. Seema was on the point of giving in, but something in her was also determined to see it through. On the final day of the third week of this battle of nerves, her son gave in. He stepped out of the shower, dressed himself in a fresh set of clothes and headed to his classes.

To me, as an educator, Seema's story, though laced with humour, was a glimpse into what love can ask of us. It takes a certain fortitude, a warrior-spirit, to be able to take a tough stance when your heart is all but breaking. The story points to the battle of holding on and letting go that families have to constantly wage. There are no right answers to the onslaught of questions: How much should one handhold a child with special needs? When should parents let go? How can parents ensure that their children grow emotionally and physically strong, even in the face of the things they cannot do? As one mother poignantly said, 'Am I using my daughter's disability as an excuse not to let go? Sometimes, I suspect that her needing me is my form of security and that her self-reliance will create a void inside me that I cannot face.'

∽

A MOUNTAINEER AND AN ENTOMOLOGIST

When sixteen-year-old Meghana and I decided to watch a film at the local theatre, the lag between policy and execution when it comes to ease of access in public spaces for the disabled was brought home to me.

Our adventure began, quite literally, with the first step. The steep ascent into the theatre was a challenge for both of us. On the one hand, Meghana's balance was impaired by cerebral palsy. On the other, I struggled to provide support in a way that would not make her self-conscious. When we finally reached the top, she exclaimed, 'Akka, I feel like I have made it to Sabrimala!' At the popcorn counter, the staff were patient as they deciphered her speech and guided her through the various choices. The smile on her face, as she balanced a tub of hot buttered popcorn, was priceless. As we navigated the narrow passages to our seats, people exchanged glances, some tittered and others simply gawked. Self-conscious at first, once the film began, Meghana was a teenager swooning at the sight of her hero and giggling at the antics on screen. After the movie was over, we had to navigate the restroom—a nightmare in itself. But none of this put off Meghana, who summed up her experience thus: 'I feel so happy, akka. I should go out more often.'

∽

Each time a student enters my class, I feel the flutter of a thousand butterflies in my gut. Even as I look forward to exploring a new mind, certain doubts persist. Will I be able to connect with the student? Will we make that journey together?

Neeraj walks into the assessment room. Shoulders hunched, eyes downcast, he has the air of a soldier who has already lost the battle. Quietly, he slips into the chair and reaches out for a pencil.

'Let us go to the garden,' I suggest. He looks surprised but follows without a word. We walk into the sunshine, feeling the grass beneath our feet. Spotting a beetle, he moves closer to inspect it. For the next ten minutes, I am treated to a lecture on the characteristics of the insect. He is an encyclopaedia of information on it and is amused at the extent of my ignorance.

Out of nowhere, he looks at me and says, 'I suck at writing and spelling.' The sudden outburst relaxes him.

'Let's find out why, shall we?' I ask.

He holds my hand as we open the door to the classroom.

BOOK SEVEN

You Expert Woman, You

Interleaved Stories

K. Srilata

Mynah Hands, Flying Fingers

Brick-like and relentless, it fell. On the window panes and on the roof. On Muniya's heart until the soaking wetness grew unbearable, this first rain of the season. In the next room, her parents were arguing, their voices rising above the rain, about whether or not they should visit Kausalya paatti, Ranjit's grandmother.

'She is in the ICU, for heaven's sake!' Baba was saying. 'What's the fucking point?'

'How can we possibly *not* go?' said Ma. 'We've been neighbours for years. They are practically family—for Muniya and me, at any rate. And Kannan and Damayanti have been so good to us.'

'You go if you feel so strongly about it. I can't come—not today. I have to get this story done or it will clean leave my mind.' Baba was a writer. A published writer who had won some of the country's top awards for writing. Everyone agreed Partho Majumdar a.k.a. Tapan was a genius.

'*I have to get this story done or it will clean leave my mind*,' Ma mimicked. 'That's all you ever think about—your precious stories. Do you ever think about Muniya? Is it enough to merely name your child after a character in a Tagore story? Is it? Do you know how fond Kausalya paatti is of her?'

'Look, Anu. I have no time for all your soppy nonsense. And why are you bringing up that name thing now? I know you never quite cared for Tagore's "*Samapti Golpo*". But I will still say it was one of his best. And don't forget, I let you have your say when it came to Mrinmoyee's *daak naam*. You were the one who picked Muniya, remember? You said she reminded you of a small bird. Anyway, that's beside the point. Let's not revisit that old argument. What I am trying to tell you is that there's no earthly use in hanging around the ICU.'

'But Mrinmoyee means made of mud! What a crazy idea to name a child that, Tapan!'

Muniya tunnelled her way back under her old quilt, pulling it all the way to the top of her head. Silence. No rain noise. No parent noise. Might as well have gone to school. When she emerged from under the quilt, the rain was still at it, pounding away on the roof, the way the letters of the alphabet pounded away at her in school. That bully, Miss Prabha, saying in front of the entire class, 'That's no way to write R and just how does one spell "snack", tell me, Mrinmoyee? What I see here is SNAKE!' Say that again and louder, Miss Prabha. Let them all hear and laugh. They know anyway—how dumb I am. Dumb is a word I can spell. D ... U ... M ... B. With a B at the end. There!

'I am off then.'

'Take Muniya with you.'

'A hospital is no place for a child. You know that as well as I do.'

'For fuck's sake, I can't work with her around. You know that, Anu.'

'Well, you will just have to find a way to deal with that, won't you, Tapan darling.'

Take me with you, Ma. I don't want to stay here with Baba. Can't you see? He doesn't want me here. Take me with you. I want to see Kausalya paatti too.

But in the end, Ma never went. She stayed home sullenly, refusing even to watch the rain which was slowly easing up and had become a gentle drumming with a distinct beat. For lunch, they had fish fry and dal rice. Muniya's favourite meal. But the child ate listlessly, her mind jumping from one thing to another—Miss Prabha, Ma and Baba's quarrels, poor Kausalya paatti. She was helping Ma clear the table when the call came. It was Kannan uncle calling from the hospital to say Kausalya paatti had passed away. The woman with mynah hands was no more. She had chosen to go on a day of glorious rains. They would be bringing her home soon. In the sort of tizzy that help the living cope with death, Ma made a series of phone calls and set about preparing chai. Gallons of it. Muniya looked at the large vessel of water and milk on the stove and marvelled at Ma's briskness and at the connections between grief and the making of vast quantities of tea. Kausalya paatti herself had always been a coffee drinker. Decoction coffee—thick and frothy. In fact, she had hated tea with the singular obsession of a coffee drinker. But Ma did not stop to reflect on the irony of this. In any case, she was making chai for the living.

Kausalya paatti had been born deaf. Over the years, her hands had evolved a syntactically perfect bird-wing language, a language all her own, which those close to her understood perfectly. If Kausalya paatti felt that the dosa her daughter-in-law served her for evening tiffin was not hot enough, the mynahs would complain bitterly. 'Paatti says her dosa is not hot enough,' Ranjit and Muniya would chorus.

'I serve it to her right off the pan and the old woman still complains,' Damayanti aunty would mutter under her breath. But for all that, she loved Kausalya paatti.

Then there was the day when Ranjit's father, Kannan uncle, had climbed a ladder to retrieve something from the loft. Half way up, he had been overcome by vertigo and had had to be helped down. Kausalya paatti had watched this scene intently. Afterwards, she had done a perfect imitation of her son climbing the ladder for the benefit of friends and neighbours. Grabbing at an imaginary ladder, placing one foot on the rung below and the other on the one above, looking downwards with eyes that pleaded, 'Help! I am feeling dizzy!' What a perfect mime artist paatti had been!

Muniya thought of those hands now, moving swiftly and gracefully through the air like a pair of mynahs, saying what they had to say. If Kausalya paatti was dead, it meant her hands were too. Those two mynahs were dead.

Muniya and Ranjit had been born on the exact same day. November babies, both. Born on a rainy day like this. They had grown up together, been admitted to the same school, the same section even. St Patrick's Academy was a neighbourhood school run by nuns in long white habits with strong, hateful hands. Nuns who believed that the only reason some children did not write was because they were cussed and stubborn, and that the only way to get them to write was to rap them on the knuckles. Ranjit had never once been rapped on his knuckles. But that was because he had his head screwed on right and was writing whole sentences by the time he was in first grade. Muniya had been rapped on her knuckles more times than she cared to remember. She was a bad, cussed, stubborn girl and fully deserved it. Ranjit sat with the boys on one side of the classroom. The law of the school dictated that boys and girls could not speak to each other and so he did not speak to Muniya. But back home, the equations changed. Back home, Ranjit of the dextrous fingers helped Muniya with her homework and lent her his notes. Back home, Ranjit, unlike the other kids in their apartment, was squarely on her side. His hands, unlike Kausalya paatti's, were well-nourished and fleshy. More like a pair of pond herons than mynahs. He used them to chat with Kausalya paatti.

One day, when her fingers started to cooperate, Muniya hoped to write Kausalya paatti's story.

When it had become clear that Muniya could not write very well, that no amount of bullying by the likes of Miss Prabha was going to do the trick, she sank into a deep, waterless well. DUMB dumb. With a 'b' at the end. There was no way she was going to learn to write. And there was no point trying. She would just wait it out until ... 'Until the school throws you out, what else? Must you be so difficult, Muniya? Can't you get those fingers of yours to hold a pencil the right way—like this?' The anguish in Ma's voice—that was another thing Muniya had grown used to. Even though, at first, it had hurt more than her own anguish, more even than her own fingers after she had tried and failed to hold the pencil right.

They brought Kausalya paatti home in the brick-like rain, all wrapped in a white hospital bed sheet, her mynah hands hidden from view and finally at rest. Damayanti aunty and Kannan uncle looked puffy-eyed and worn out. Ranjit looked as if he had been sitting on his tears. That was because he was a boy. Boys didn't cry. Only girls did. But Muniya never cried. Not even when Sister Priscilla rapped her on her knuckles. Muniya snuck up to Ma and peeked at the body, for that is what Kausalya paatti was now—a body. Someone was talking about her—about its—eyes. Apparently, its eyes had been removed and donated to a blind girl. It had been its—her—wish. Kausalya paatti's wish. Sandwiched between a press of adults, Muniya tried long and hard to get a glimpse of those mynahs. But that was not to be. They were weighed down by rose garlands. Ma barked at her to get out of the way. She was running around, serving everyone chai, her long hair flying behind her. What would Kausalya paatti have said about the chai?

That night, as Muniya lay beside Ma, she asked, 'Did Paatti not want her hands to be donated, Ma?'

'Why? What an idea!' exclaimed Ma.

'I would have liked them,' said Muniya, after a while. But Ma had drifted into a deep sleep and was no longer listening. All night long, Muniya dreamt of Paatti's mynahs perched on her fingers, guiding them to write. First, the alphabets. And then, the words. And then, slowly, those sentences like snakes. Those long, looong sentences.

All the while, Sister Priscilla bending over her, a sweet smile on her lips. 'Good girl, Mrinmoyee! See, you can be a good girl too, if you try! Just look at your fingers flying!'

Things Not Known to Happen

Ma, as usual, was trying to make up. Muniya knew the signs only too well. There was a dreadful sameness to these episodes. First, Ma would fly into a rage. You couldn't really blame her for it because, mostly, it *was* Muniya's doing. It was Muniya who gave Ma all this grief. Small and big doses of grief on a daily basis. By not working hard enough. By not doing enough. Or, simply, by not being enough. *Why can't you be like the others, Muniya? Is it so damn hard?* Not that Ma ever spoke those words out aloud. But Muniya knew they were buzzing around inside her head. Those words were the background noise they lived with. From time to time, this background noise would erupt into the volcanic spewing of Ma's temper. At such times, Ma was like a woman possessed. Nothing could stop the torrent of words. *You will be the death of me. You don't love your Ma. If you did, would you do this to me? How many hours I spent explaining that lesson to you? Did you even listen? You are not dumb. I know that. But does the world know that? No! They think you are stupid. Stupid. Heard that? I don't want them to think that of you. Ever. Because you are not! Heard that? But if you refuse to listen to me, if you insist on being lazy and difficult and stubborn ... Stubborn child. That's what you are. Stubborn. Won't listen. Won't do as I say. Did I not tell you a million times to check your work? To do the long answers properly? To list out the points on the margins before you begin writing? To check and double check your spellings? But no. You can't be bothered, can you? Just look at this answer. Every single word misspelt. Is there no end to your carelessness, Muniya? Stubborn girl. Don't you care about me at all? Don't you?*

The spewing would continue for a while, until Ma ran out of energy. Sometimes, one long spewing session would be followed by a series of tiny bursts. And then, quite suddenly, as though some switch had been turned off in her head, Ma would slump in her chair. Seconds later, she would begin purring like a kitten. She would hug Muniya for no reason, kiss her fiercely on both cheeks several times. Again, for no reason. If this happened on a weekend, she would take Muniya to the mall and buy her something fancy or to the movies (things Ma otherwise never did, for, in her world, these came under the heading 'waste of time' or 'time that could be better spent teaching Muniya').

When Ma was in one of those moods, there was nothing Muniya or anyone else could do. She would work on autopilot. Baba would shut himself up in his study to 'write'. Baba was like that—head in the sand in times of trouble. Lakshmi, their maid, would skunk in and out timidly, trying her best to stop the dishes from clattering, throwing a sympathetic glance at Muniya now and then.

The first time Ma turned into an active volcano, Muniya had been terrified. She had failed her social science exam. Ingloriously. Grand total score: 1/50. Ma had spent hours coaching her for it, setting mock papers that Muniya had fared reasonably well on. But the moment the teacher had handed her the question paper, she had gone and lost her nerve. Cold and clammy hands, vision all blurry and brain all packed up. Muniya had had one of her infamous word-emptiness attacks. An hour later, she had handed in her answer sheet, mostly blank, except for a one-mark multiple-choice question on what the word 'indigo' in the 'indigo rebellion' meant. The options given were: a. flight, b. a car model, c. a colour and d. a food crop. Muniya had ticked option c. The previous day, Ma had shown her a duppatta of hers that was dyed indigo. That visual anchor must have helped with the recall.

All things considered, Ma had been perfectly justified in erupting. That first time, Muniya had shrunk into herself and wept silently. Over the years, in the face of more volcanic episodes, Muniya had come to understand that Ma's spewing would last only a short while. She would always always regret it and would end up most contrite. (Immediately afterwards, in fact. Kisses, cuddles and silly little gifts would follow.) Muniya saw that the spewing came from a place of deep love and deep despair, that it couldn't be helped. Better the volcano than no Ma, she reasoned to herself. And so Muniya forgave and forgot. Until the next eruption. And then again, she forgave and forgot.

Ma, her Ma, had been a beautiful woman once. Muniya had seen pictures of her from before the time she was born. Pictures in which Ma had flowing, jet-black hair, a face devoid of wrinkles, no shadows under her eyes. Pictures in which Ma was not spewing or slumped in her chair. Muniya had also seen pictures of herself as a baby, Ma and Baba holding her, their faces happy and smiling.

Muniya thought now of those pictures. There would be other pictures in the future, she told herself. Pictures of herself done with school, all grown up and working at some posh office. Pictures, once again, of Ma with flowing, jet-black hair, a face devoid of wrinkles, no shadows under her eyes. Yes. These pictures were entirely possible. Even though nothing about the present moment seemed to suggest they were. Things not known to happen could happen too. Alongside things that were known to happen. The only thing to be done was to wait it out. Inside this large, warm, temporary space of a mother's contrite hug.

You Expert Woman, You

It wasn't as though the expert was unkind. And yet, what she said was delivered like an insult. It was the tone she used with Ma. Muniya, who was familiar with all manner of insults, was a mistress of tone. She could smell them coming her way, the subtle ones and the not-so subtle ones: the Sister Priscilla insult (ten sharp raps on her knuckles with a cane), the neighbour aunty Shanta insult (an over-bright smile that had *I am broad-minded* plastered all over it), the Baba insult (*do I really have a daughter?*), the Liz insult (*but this is suuper easy, Muniya, I didn't even have to study it!*). Every day, she waited for these insults to descend on her thin, small body, on her baby soul and every day, she looked as though she didn't give a damn. *So what? So what? So what?*

And yet, this woman and her questions, her over-soft, deadly serious voice ... They couldn't not give a damn— she and Ma. She was an 'expert', Ma had explained to her beforehand. She would run some simple tests on Muniya and then ... And then what? And then, well, all would be well. *But what's the matter with me, Ma?* was the question stuck in Muniya's throat. That question had been stuck down there ever since that terrible meeting with the principal of St Patrick's. Muniya could have sworn she had heard the woman say, 'We don't want children like you.' But the fact of the matter was that the principal had spoken over her head to Ma. 'We can't teach children like her, Mrs Mukherjee. It is best you find another place for her. We are sorry, Mrs Mukherjee. She doesn't seem to want to learn. There may be other schools willing to take her.'

A week before, at the school annual day event, Liz had been awarded the merit prize. All sorts of kids had got all sorts of prizes or, at the very least, certificates, and Muniya had clapped for each one of them. It was the thing to do, after all. But no one had clapped for her when she had got her certificate.

Tell me about the day she was born, Mrs Mukherjee.

She was a preemie. Tiny enough to fit in my palm.

Ma smiles at me. We are in this together.

It was a day like any other. Except for the rains. Oh, how it rained! It was a struggle to get to hospital ...

And the labour pains? Where they very intense? Did they last long?

Yes. Yes, they did.

So, I was always trouble.

And then?

They had to suction her out.

Was there, for instance, a lack of oxygen at any point in the process?

No. At least they didn't say so.

Mrs Mukherjee, did she cry when she was born?

Oh yes! Oh yes!

At once?

Yes, oh yes!

Now, think carefully. Did she latch on at once?

I beg your pardon?

Did she latch on, you know, did she feed properly, at birth?

Yes. Yes, she did. Muniya, I mean Mrinmoyee, was a real hungry baby. She ...

Did she roll over, crawl, sit up, all at the right time?

Mmmm ...

Did I, Ma?

Yes, I suppose she did. I can't remember now. She seemed okay. She was a lovely ...

Try and remember, Mrs Mukherjee.

Well, I remember my mother saying she was late turning over. Other than that, she was perf—

Go ahead, say it Ma. Other than that, she was perfect. A perfect baby. I was a perfect baby. A lovely baby. Hear that, you expert woman, you?

When did she start to walk?

One year and two months. Is that late? It is, isn't it?

When did she start to talk?

She was late talking.

It is alright, Ma. Don't give up the fight.

She was two when she spoke her first words. My mother was worried.

That is an indication, Mrs Mukherjee.

Of what? Of what?

Have you and your husband ever struggled with any learning disabilities? Any dyslexia in the family?

No. No, we haven't. Struggled, I mean. We were alright, I suppose, my husband and I. He is a writer, in fact, and I ...

Does she have friends?

Yes. Yes. There's a boy next door—Ranjit—she is ... they are best friends. They grew up together. Even went to school ...

How about pencil grip?

Muniya ... Mrinmoyee was amazing in every way. But she never could manage to hold the pencil the right way. I tried everything. Everything.

Fine motor control issues there, certainly.

She has great conceptual clarity. Always had. She is a bright kid.

She struggled in school, didn't she?

Yes...yes. I am afraid she did.

I was awarded a transfer certificate. The other kids, they got other sorts of certificates. Ma's eyes that day were puffy and red.

The expert woman looks at me.

'Come here, child,' she says. *I go to her, wishing I was a bird, wishing I could fly out the window.*

The expert woman hands me a pencil. Let us see you holding this, she says. I do as I am told. It is a Flora pencil with pretty pink flowers on it. I hate Flora pencils. In fact, I hate all pencils.

'Not like that,' she says. 'Like this, see?'

I do as I am told.

'Write your name,' she says.

I write Mrinmoyee. I can do that. I can write my name, expert woman, you. I am not dumb. My fingers have slipped back to the former position. The wrong position. The expert woman takes my hand in hers and positions the fingers correctly once again. 'Like this, child.'

She looks at Ma, who is looking worried, and whips out a pad.

'Make an appointment with the OT—Geetha. She deals with fine motor control issues. It may help.'

What's OT?

'Will she be alright, ma'am?' I have never heard my mother call anyone 'ma'am' before. No, actually, I have. Just that one time in the principal's office at St Patrick's. (*Please, ma'am. Won't you reconsider? Just give my daughter one more chance.*)

'That depends, Mrs Mukherjee. That depends. On her. On you. Child, you must work very very hard. Alright? Do whatever the OT tells you to do.'

I nod. If I do what the OT tells me to do, will I turn into

Liz? Will they give me the merit prize? I want to ask. But this question too sticks in my throat.

On the way home, Ma treats me and herself to an ice cream. I am not sure why, though. There is no reason to celebrate. 'OT' did not sound like a happy or kind word.

Ma is a messy eater. She has blobs of ice cream all over her kurta.

'Fine motor control issues,' she murmurs, unhappy-silly-drunk on ice cream. 'And who doesn't have them.' A chocolate blob runs down the corner of her mouth. And me, I am a bird who has flown out the window of the expert woman's room. I am a girl with mynah hands, dexterous and capable of things the expert woman knows nothing of.

Rainbow Loom Bracelet

It had seemed to her, for the longest time, that others knew things she didn't. That they were born knowing those things. And that she, Muniya, had been born *not* knowing them. That she was missing some vital part. So, it didn't appear likely that she would make it to the happy garden, the one which the other children inhabited. But Ma, ever hopeful, had moved her, after the meeting with that expert woman, out of St Patrick's into Riverstone, which they said was an *inclusive* school. And at first—with all its fanciness—it did appear as though it was. And that boy, Jayanth, who mostly didn't speak, was there as well—in the same class as Muniya, in fact. And if it worked for him, it would surely work for Muniya. But, in the end, Riverstone had come a cropper too and Ma had had to get her out of that and into this new place. And this was to be Muniya's happy garden—for this place was not a school. Muniya knew that in her bones. She was, all said and done, a school veteran, a battle-scarred warrior. She knew what school was and what it wasn't. In school, one did proper subjects such as math, history and science. In this place, one did not. Not to the same torturous degree at any rate. Muniya's stomach had hurt all the time when she was at St Patrick's. Not even the fact that Ranjit was in the same class as her had helped. Muniya's stomach had hurt much of the time she was at Riverstone too, notwithstanding its fanciness, its air of 'every kind of child is welcome here' (what a lie!). She thought often of Kausalya paatti's mynah hands. How she missed them! The only happy thing about Riverstone, in fact, had been Jayanth—the boy who never spoke—who, before he actually ventured to speak to her, wrote her these little notes. Notes that said 'I love you' and 'You will be alright' and 'My name is Yellow Leaf though everyone here calls me Jayanth'. Notes written in such a poor hand she could barely read them. She wrote him back a note too once: 'My name is Muniya though everyone here calls me Mrinmoyee. And you are nice.' And then, soon after that, she had showed him her hiding place, the place where she ate her lunch. It was there that he had kissed her and they had been caught out. That had been the end of Riverstone for her. For Jayanth too. Riverstone would not tolerate 'inappropriate behaviour', the principal had declared, and Ma had melted into tears. Oh! The shame of it all, overlaying all the other kinds of shame ... Where was Jayanth now? Had he started to speak to other people? How she missed him! It had been her fault entirely. She should never have shown him that secret lunch place of hers.

In this new place, Muniya's stomach did not hurt. There was one downside, though. You could get bored out of your skull doing all the things they told you to.

They spent the first half of the day rolling on the floor and breathing in and out through alternate nostrils. Occasionally, they got to walk around the playground on tiptoe, which was a treat, relatively speaking. There were fancy names for all the stuff they were made to do but Muniya couldn't say them.

The adults in charge of them were not unfriendly. They were just unimaginative and frazzled. They flapped about like penguins as they persuaded them to get on with it. It was Sameeha who had first observed their resemblance to penguins. She had been admitted to the place a few months after Muniya. There were ten of them, in all. Six boys, two other girls who were twins and kept to themselves, Sameeha and Muniya.

Sameeha's skin was like ebony and her hair, frizzy beyond belief, reminded Muniya of the pine trees up in the hills of Kodaikanal. Baba used to go there sometimes so he could write in peace—without her and Ma getting in the way. Baba, Ma and Muniya lived in a small two-bedroom apartment and Baba always complained he had no space in which to think or write. Ma said that was too bad, this was all they had and if he didn't like it, why didn't he go out and get himself a proper job. Ma worked as a teacher in a school for posh kids. She had, at one point, tried to get Muniya into that school but the school would have nothing to do with a child like Muniya. Liza, rosy-cheeked and smart as they come, could have gotten into that school had she wanted to. But then, Liza was a normal child. Muniya, who knew it was wrong to hate people, could not help hating Liza. Liza, super-smart Liza from St Patrick's, was miles ahead of her, always would be. There was no question of catching up. Not ever.

One way in which you could think of Sameeha was that she was the antonym of Liza. This said, however, ten Lizas put together could not beat Sameeha when it came to certain things. Sameeha had the wildest imagination. 'Look! They are like penguins!' she had declared, and they had giggled uncontrollably. They had become soul sisters soon after that, rolling on the floor together, breathing through alternate nostrils in hysterical unison and closely examining each other's moles. In short, they had fun, which was orthogonal to the vision of the place, but who cared. The penguins had too much on their plate. Ten kids with odd minds and this included a boy who peed in his pants just for larks, lazy ayahs who rolled their hips as they walked, a one-eyed watchman who snored on the job and the heat ... Really, what could you do with the bunch of them and in that heat?

One hot summer afternoon, Muniya had kissed Sameeha and they had both giggled. What followed were rainbow loom bands made on the sly when the penguins were otherwise occupied. Sameeha's mother had bought her a kit and she had sneaked it into the place. They fashioned the bands over lunch—the two of them, their strong little hands moving rapidly against time. When the penguins called out to them, they took a whole minute to gaze at the amazing twirls they had created, fragile, shot through with colour, heartbreakingly beautiful.

A year and a half after Sameeha had sneaked in her first rainbow loom kit, Muniya had eventually made it to almost-normal. At least in the eyes of Ma, who had pulled her out of the place in a grand burst of energy and got her admitted to a new school in the neighbourhood desperate for students and which claimed to have a special educator on its staff. The only not-so-nice thing was that Muniya would be placed in a grade meant for younger children. But that was alright, Ma said. It would be easier on her Muniya. Yes, Muniya could do it. Hopefully. Fingers crossed. If all went well.

Ma had more grey hair than black and this was how it had been for a long time. Though no one had ever said so, Muniya was sure this had to do with her. Sameeha's Ma was the same. All the mothers of the children in that place had more grey hair than black. That was just the way it was. And one never saw the fathers. That too was just the way it was. The children owed their mothers. Muniya owed Ma.

And partly for that reason, and partly because she had no choice, she had had to make that terrifying leap. For Normal stood on the other side of the canyon. She would be safe inside that happy garden *if* she made the effort. If all went well, Ma's hair would become pitch black like Liza's mother's. *Leap, Muniya, leap. Don't look back. Enter the happy garden. Become exactly like the others.*

On her last day in that place Sameeha had made her a rainbow loom bracelet. It was a bracelet to die for. This one had all the rainbow colours.

Muniya slipped the little rainbow quietly around her wrist. She would never ever take this off. *Never ever.* Not even if the penguins in her new school insisted.

'Bye Sameeha! See you soon!' Trite, hollow words. It was only afterwards that she had thought of the right words to say. *Leap, Sameeha, leap. Don't look back. Follow me to the happy garden. Together, let us become exactly like the others.*

Afterword

Writers, we know, grow as they write. And the converse is equally true. Writing grows, deepens, expands, in tandem with the writer. I am not the same person going into this book as I am coming out. The book too has changed contours, expanded outwards. It is as though many doors have been thrown open and all at the same time.

This is an open-ended story. The people in *This Kind of Child* will continue to grow, find other ways to inhabit the world. Their stories recorded here will become history, a history that matters. It is entirely possible that when the people in this book revisit their narratives, they will wonder at their old selves. Maybe, they will marvel at how far afield they have travelled. And then, of course, from the time I started working on this book to now, the world has seen a pandemic. We are still not sure what the impact of that has been on people with disabilities. How many of them have lost jobs? What impact has 'work from home', school closures, the lack of access to medical services, therapy and special education, the deaths of loved ones and just the sheer isolation of these times had on them? What impact has all of this had on the people in this book? I wonder and I worry.

This Kind of Child is an entire community of people— people who may not know each other but who share in the same larger conversation and are present here—alongside each other. They are asking the question we are all asking ourselves: What does it mean to live in this body, in this mind and navigate the world?

Acknowledgements

This book owes its existence to the generosity of so many. To all the people who are part of its fabric, thank you. Thank you for the gift of your time, thank you for trusting me with your stories, thank you for staying the course.

Thanks to Karthika V.K. for believing in the story I set out to tell, for her unwavering commitment to it. To Sonia, Saurabh and all the wonderful people at Westland for the love and the careful attention they gave to this book, my deepest gratitude.

Thanks to my mother Vatsala, to Mani, Aniruddha and Ananya. Their presence illumines this book.

And thank you to my chosen family—friends too numerous to name—but you know who you are. Thank you for your support and for your love.